AF352401

Choline, Phospholipids, Health, and Disease

Editors

Steven H. Zeisel
University of North Carolina at Chapel Hill
Chapel Hill, North Carolina

Bernard F. Szuhaj
Central Soya Company, Inc.
Fort Wayne, Indiana

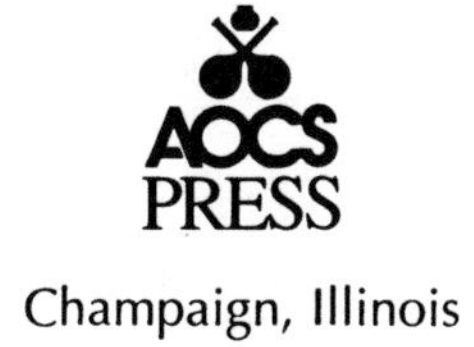

AOCS PRESS

Champaign, Illinois

Library of Congress Cataloging-in-Publication Data
Choline, phospholipids, health, and disease / editors, Steven H.
   Zeisel, Bernard F. Szuhaj.
      p. cm.
   Proceedings of the 7th International Congress on Phospholipids,
held in Brussels, Sept. 1996.
   Includes bibliographical references and index.
   ISBN 0-935315-86-1 (alk. paper)
   1. Phospholipids—Physiological effect—Congresses. 2. Choline—
Physiological effect—Congresses. 3. Phospholipids—
Pathophysiology—Congresses. 4. Choline—Pathophysiology—
Congresses. I. Zeisel, Steven H. II. Szuhaj, Bernard F.
III. American Oil Chemists' Society. IV. International Colloquium
on Phospholipids (7th : 1996 : Brussels, Belgium)
   [DNLM: 1. Phospholipids congresses. 2. Choline congresses. QU
93C5466 1998]
QP752.P53C48   1998
DNLM/DLC
612'.01577—dc21
for Library of Congress   98-39864
                                                      CIP

Printed in the United States of America with vegetable oil-based inks.
01 00 99 98   5 4 3 2 1

Preface

There is much interest today in the essentiality of choline (see *Dietary Reference Intakes for Thiamin, Riboflavin, Niacin, Vitamin B$_6$, Folate, Vitamin B$_{12}$, Pantothenic Acid, Biotin, and Choline,* the recent recommendations of the Institute of Medicine, National Academy of Science, USA). In anticipation of that need, a meeting was developed by the AOCS Phospholipid Division to bring the top researchers in choline and choline phospholipids together to exchange their research results and plan for new projects and programs throughout the world.

These proceedings are the result of many manhours put together to update the nutrition, health, and medical research community on the latest work being done on phospholipids in health and disease. Some of the papers were reviews and some were original research.

A number of colloquiums, symposiums, and congresses have been held since 1980 that covered Lecithin and Phospholipids that resulted in books on technological, biological, therapeutic, biochemical, pharmaceutical, and analytical considerations. The 7th International Congress on Phospholipids held in Brussels, BG September 1996 was dedicated to Choline, Phospholipids, Health, and Disease. The program was sponsored by the AOCS Phospholipid Division and organized by Bernard F. Szuhaj. Steven H. Zeisel was the Technical Chairman and put the tremendous program together. Time was well spent during this three-day meeting with over 100 participants and dozens of posters. Many new and old friends shared their research on phospholipids. This book will give the reader some insight on what was presented at this Congress.

Some of the papers covered the importance of homocystein in atherosclerosis, apoptosis, cell signaling, platelet activation, dietary choline, and pregnancy, just to name a few chapters in these proceedings. All papers have been peer reviewed and are an excellent additon to any research library.

Much thanks goes to the AOCS for sponsoring the program and to the speakers who took the time to do the research, write the manuscripts, and present the papers.

Steven H. Zeisel
Bernard F. Szuhaj

Acknowledgments

We would like to thank the AOCS staff for their assistance in coordinating this Congress in Brussels, especially Mary Belding. Many hours were spent making this a smooth and organized conference.

We would also like to thank the companies that provided monetary support for the speaker funds. These companies included:

Archer Daniels Midland, Decatur, Illinois
Avanti Polar Lipids, Inc., Alabaster, Alabama
Central Soya Company Incorporated, Fort Wayne, Indiana
Lucas Meyer GmbH, Hamburg, Germany
Nattermann Phospholipid GmbH, Cologne, Germany
N.V. Vamo Mills Protein & Lecithin Division, Belgium
Riceland Foods, Little Rock, Arkansas

Special thanks go to Randy Zigmont for tracking the finances, and for his enthusiasm for this project. Final thanks go to Joan Fisher for her support and efforts on the Congress and other AOCS/ILPS activities.

Contents

Preface...iii

Acknowledgments...iv

Chapter 1   Sphingomyelin and Other Sphingomyelin Metabolites
in Cell Signaling and Disease...1
Eva-Maria Schmelz, Mariana Nikolova-Karakashian,
Elaine Wang, and Alfred H. Merrill, Jr.

Chapter 2   Choline Phospholipids and Cell Suicide 11
Chi-Liang E. Yen and Steven H. Zeisel

Chapter 3   Phosphatidylethanolamine *N*-Methyltransferase: An
Unexpected Regulator of Hepatocyte Cell Division.................23
Dennis E. Vance, Zheng Cui, Martin Houweling,
Christopher J. Walkey, and Luciana Tessitore

Chapter 4   Antineoplastic Phospholipids Inhibit
Phosphatidylcholine Biosynthesis 30
Suzanne Jackowski and Kevin Boggs

Chapter 5   Phosphoinositides, Phospholipase D,
and Membrane Trafficking 45
Mordechai Liscovitch

Chapter 6   Phosphatidylserine as a Signal for Recognition
and Phagocytosis: The Proteins Involved 57
Robert A. Schlegel, Stephen Krahling, Allison J. Christie,
and Patrick Williamson

Chapter 7   Neurochemical Effects of Altered Prenatal Choline
Availability in Rats 69
Jan Krzysztof Blusztajn, Thomas Holler,
Jennifer Marie Cermak, and Darrell A. Jackson

Chapter 8   Origin of Axonal Lipids in Rat Sympathetic Neurons.............80
Jean E. Vance, Elena Posse de Chaves, Antonio E. Rusiñol,
Robert B. Campenot, Miguel Bussiere, and Dennis E. Vance

Chapter 9   Lowe Syndrome: A Human Inborn Error
of Phosphatidylinositol Metabolism..92
Sharon F. Suchy and Robert L. Nussbaum

Chapter 10 Alterations in Myocardial Phospholipid Metabolism
During Myocardial Ischemia..100
Richard W. Gross

Chapter 11 An Isoform of Intracellular Platelet-Activating Factor
(PAF) Acetylhydrolase and Its Relationship
to Miller-Dieker Syndrome 109
Hiroyuki Arai, Mitsuharu Hattori, Junken Aoki,
and Keizo Inoue

Chapter 12   Homocysteine and Vascular Disease: The Role
             of Folate, Choline, and Lipoproteins
             in Homocysteine Metabolism 117
             Kilmer S. McCully

Chapter 13   Choline and Choline Esters as Required Nutrients
             During Pregnancy and Lactation 131
             Steven H. Zeisel

             List of Attendees 143

             Index 144

Meeting Abstracts

Phospholipids: Growth, Death, and Cancer

Sphingomyelin and Other Sphingomyelin Metabolites in Cell Signaling and Disease. Alfred Merrill, Jr., Mariana Nikolova-Karakashian, Eva-Maria Schmelz, and Elaine Wang, Emory University School of Medicine, Department of Biochemistry, Atlanta, GA 30322-3050 USA.

Sphingomyelin and its metobolites (ceramide, sphingosine, sphingosine 1-phosphate, and sphingosylphosphorylcholine) are potent modulators of cell growth, differentiation, diverse cell behaviors, and program cell death. Many studies have focused on the involvement of these bioactive compounds as the "second messengers" for a given agonist; however, presumption is that a given agonist induces the formation of a single sphingolipid "signal"—for example, ceramide production from sphingomyelin turnover induced by cytokines. We have found several systems in which changes in multiple sphingolipids are likely to be involved in both normal and abnormal cell regulation. In rat hepatocytes, ≥ 5 ng/mL of interleukin-1β (IL-1β) induces sphingomyelin turnover and ceramide accumulation; whereas, addition of lower levels of IL-1β also activate ceramidase and there is little change in ceramide despite significant hydrolysis of sphingomyelin. This bimodal response mirrors the differential effects of IL-1β and sphingolipids on the expression of two acute phase proteins (CYP2C11 versus α_1-acid glycoprotein). Naturally occurring inhibitors of sphingolipid metabolism (fumonisins) inhibit ceramide synthase, thereby blocking complex sphingolipid synthesis and accumulation of sphinganine (and sometimes sphingosine). Although free sphingoid bases are highly cytotoxic and may account for the cytotoxicity of fumonisins; we have found that fumonisins also divert sphinganine and sphingosine to the 1-phosphates and N-acetyl-derivatives; therefore these bioactive metabolites might also play a role in pathogenesis. In other studies, we are exploring the role of sphingolipids in the behavior of colonic cells in culture (HT-29 cells) and animals fed dietary sphingolipids after administration of 1,2-dimethylhydrazine to induce aberrant colonic crypt foci and adenocarcinomas. Here, too, endogenous and exogenous sphingolipids induce profound changes in cell behavior with provocative structure/function relationships. Although the effects of sphingosine and ceramide are difficult to sort out because these compounds are metabolically interconverted, such studies are aided by naturally occurring inhibitors of ceramide synthase (i.e., fumonisins). All together, these studies underscore the diverse and complex roles of sphingolipids as second messengers, mediators of the action of toxins, and as potentially beneficial components of the diet.

Ceramide and Cell Suicide Pathways. Martin Krönke, University of Kiel, Institute of Immunology, Brunswiker Str. 4, 24105 Kiel, Germany.

Tumor necrosis factor (TNF) is a potent mediator of inflammation which has been implicated in the pathogenesis of devastating clinical syndromes including septic shock. TNF elicits biological effects through two distinct cell surface receptors p55 (TNF-R55) and p75 (TNF-R75). A recently identified cytoplasmic region on

TNF-55, designated "death domain," seems to play a major role in TNF cytotoxicity. A death domain–responsive phosphatidylcholine specific phospholipase C (PC-PLC) is shown to mediate not only *in vitro* cytotoxicity but also proinflammatory effects in animal models. So far, phospholipase A2 (PLA2) has been mostly incriminated to mediate TNF cytotoxicity; however, the mechanism of PLA2-induced remained cytotoxicity obscure. By structure function analysis of TNF-R55, it is shown that activation of PLA2 does not correlate with death domain function. Instead a signaling pathway involving a sequential activation of PC-PLC and an endosomal acid sphingomyelinase (A-SMase) appear to be essential players in the cytotoxin action of TNF. TRADD, a TNF-R55–associated protein, itself contains a death domain and signals also for activation of PC-PLC. Furthermore, D609, a specific inhibitor of PC-PLC, completely blocks TNF cytotoxicity on L929 and Wehi 164 cells. Clearly, *in vitro* cytotoxic effects of PC-PLC are not necessarily tantamount to pathophysiological effects of TNF *in vivo*. Intriguingly, D609 is effective *in vivo*. In TNF-treated mice, D-609 inhibits adhesion molecule expression by endothelial cells, monoclear infiltration of the lung and eventually lethality. In shock models, D609 proved protective. when mice were challenged with lethal doses of LPS or superantigenes like SEB. C-type phospholipase such as PC-PLC and A-SMase seem to play important roles in the pathogenic action of TNF and may serve as novel targets for the development of anti-inflammatory drugs.

Choline Phospholipids and Cell Suicide Pathways. Steven H. Zeisel, Craig D. Albright, Angelica Vrablic, and Rudolf I. Salganik. University of North Carolina, Department of Nutrition, CB #7400, McGavran-Greenberg, Chapel Hill, NC 27599-7400 USA.

Immortalized CWSV-1 rat hepatocytes, in which p53 protein is inactivated by SV40 large T antigen, had increased numbers of cells with strand breaks in genomic DNA (Terminal dUTP End Labeling) when grown in 0 μM choline (67–73% of cells) than when grown in 70 μM choline (2–3% of cells). Internucleosomal fragmentation of DNA (DNA ladders) was detected in cell growth with 5 μM and 0 μM choline for 72 h. Cells treated with 0 or 5 μM choline exhibited a high incidence of apoptosis (apoptotic bodies were seen in 55–75% of cells; 67–73% had DNA strand breaks). p53 protein is thought to be indispensable for the induction of apoptosis by most triggers. Western blot analysis showed that p53 in the nucleus of cells was detected in direct association with SV40 T-antigen, and was therefore likely to be inactivated. CWSV1 cells were resistant to γ-irradiation, also suggesting p53 was inactivated. The novel anti cancer drug 1-*O*-octadecyl-2-*O*-methyl-rac-glycero-3-phosphocholine inhibits the CDP-choline pathway of phosphatidylcholine synthesis. Hepatocytes treated with this drug die by apoptosis. We conclude that choline deficiency kills CWSV-1 hepatocytes in culture by inducing apoptosis via what may be a p53-independent process, and that this process may occur because phosphatidylcholine synthesis has been perturbed. In the liver of rats fed a choline deficient (CD) diet for six weeks classical apoptotic bodies were detected in 0.28 ± 0.04 percent of hepatocytes compared to 0.096 ± 0.006 percent of hepatocytes in control rats fed a choline sufficient (CS) diet. In CD animals, DNA fragmentation characteristic of an apoptotic process was detected using digoxigenin-11-dUTP and a TUNEL method in 29.7 ± 9.0 percent of hepatocytes scattered throughout the liver. In CS controls, DNA strand breaks were detected only in 0.38 ± 0.19 percent of hepatocytes, mostly in cells near the terminal hepatic vein. We found that feeding a CD diet is not associated with the nuclear localization of p53 protein in hepatocytes. Thus it is possible that CD triggers a p53-independent apoptosis pathway in rat hepatocytes. TGFβ1 protein and the related p27^{Kip1} checkpoint protein are known to function independently of p53. The data presented show that the vast majority of hepatocytes in CD liver express high levels of TGFβ1 protein as well as TGFβ1 receptor types I and II. Expression of p27^{Kip1} protein, which may link TGFβ1 expression to cell cycle arrest and apoptosis, showed a ten-fold increase in CD hepatocytes (4.1 ± 1.1 vs. 0.35 ± 0.04 percent in CD vs. CS). We conclude that feeding a choline deficient diet induces apoptosis in hepatocytes in rat liver. CD-triggered apoptosis appears to be mediated by TGFβ1 and related proteins independent of p53 protein.

Phosphatidylethanolamine *N*-Methyltransferase: An Unexpected Candidate Tumor Suppressor and Regulator of Hepatocyte Cell Division. Dennis E. Vance, Zheng Cui, Martin Houweling, Chris Walkey, University of Alberta, Lipid and Lipoprotein Research Group and Department of Biochemistry, Edmonton, Alberta, Canada; Luciana Tessitore, Hospital San Luigi of Orbassano, Department of Clinical and Biological Sciences, Torino, Italy.

Phosphatidylethanolamine *N*-Methyltransferase (PEMT) occurs in two forms, PEMT1 localized to the endoplasmic reticulum and PEMT2 localized to the mitochondria-associated membrane. Expression of the cDNA for PEMT2 in McArdle rat hepatoma cells slowed the rate of cell division from 20 to 50 h. We have now found that PEMT2 is inactivated in rat liver tumors and precancerous lesions induced by chemical carcinogens. Marked decreased expression of PEMT2 occurs in the first detectable lesions and is completely absent in advanced nodules and more advanced stages of hepatic cancer. There is also a decrease in PEMT activity. In contrast, the activity of CPT:phosphocholine cytidylytransferase of the CDP-choline pathway is nearly doubled in advanced stages of hepatoma. These data define PEMT2 as a candidate tumor suppressor. Since p53, retinoblastoma protein and other suppressor proteins do not appear to play a role in liver cancer, PEMT2 is the first liver-specific tumor suppressor identified and is the first enzyme in lipid metabolism to be linked to tumor suppression. In addition, studies on liver regeneration, lead nitrate–induced hyperplasia and developmental expression, all link PEMT2 to the regulation of cell division in normal liver. In each case reduced expression of PEMT2 is associated with liver growth. Thus, PEMT2 appears to have an unexpected role in the regulation of hepatocyte cell division.

Antineoplastic Phospholipids Inhibit Phosphatidylcholine Biosynthesis. Suzanne Jackowski, St. Jude Children's Hospital, Department of Biochemistry, 332 N. Lauderdale, Memphis, TN 38105-2794 USA.

The relationship between the inhibition of phospholipid synthesis and the cytotoxic activity of antineoplastic lysophosphatidylcholine analogs was investigated in hematopoietic cell lines. Lysophosphatidylcholine (lysoPtdCho), 1-*O*-octadecyl-2-

O-methyl-*rac*-glycero-3-phosphocholine (ET-18-OCH$_3$), and hexadecyl-phosphorylcholine (HexPC) reduced the *de novo* biosynthesis of phosphatidylcholine (PtdCho) in a dose-dependent manner. The relative distribution of metabolic precursors to PtdCho indicated that inhibition occurred at the CTP:phosphocholine cytidylyltransferase (CT) step. Direct inhibition of CT enzyme activity by lysoPtdCho, ET-18-OCH$_3$, and HexPC was demonstrated *in vitro* when the soluble protein was purified from endogenous, bound lipid. LysoPtdCho was metabolized to PtdCho following cellular uptake and enabled the bypass of *de novo* biosynthesis. These data reveal lysoPtdCho as a physiological regulator of PtdCho synthesis at the CT step that is mimicked by the nonmetabolized structural analogs. Cell cycle progression of synchronized cells was impaired by treatment with ET-18-OCH$_3$ and resulted in blocks at both the G$_1$ and G$_2$ phases. Apoptosis was evident in cells blocked at either phase. Incubation of cells with exogenous lysoPtdCho in the presence of ET-18-OCH$_3$ rescued the cells from the block in G$_2$ phase and from apoptosis, resulting in viable cells with normal morphology. Treatment of a human HL60 leukemic cell line with either ET-18-OCH$_3$ or HexPC also resulted in cell death due to apoptosis, incubation with lysoPtdCho was able to overcome the cytotoxic effects of the antineoplastic drugs. These results demonstrate that inhibition of PtdCho synthesis by ET-18-OCH$_3$ or HexPC triggers apoptosis and suggest that the cellular levels of CT, the drug target, contribute to chemotherapeutic drug selectivity and dose efficacy.

Phosphoinositides, Phospholipase D, and Membrane Trafficking. Mordechai Liscovitch, The Weizmann Institute of Science, Rehovot 76100, Israel.

Receptor-dependent activation of phosphatidylcholine–specific phospholipase D (PLD) is a widespread phenomenon. A variety of neurotransmitters, hormones, growth factors, and constituents of the extracellular matrix causes a rapid and dramatic activation of PLD, indicating a role in signal transduction. The existence of multiple forms of signal-activated PLD in mammalian cells is supported by studies showing the differential subcellular localization, distinct mechanisms of activation and substrate specificities, and different chromatographic properties of putative PLD isozymes. PLD requires a lipid cofactor, phosphatidylinositol 4,5-bisphosphate (PIP$_2$). Ongoing synthesis of PIP$_2$ is essential for PLD activation by G proteins and protein kinase C. Intriguingly, both PLD and phosphoinositide kinases have been implicated in intracellular vesicular trafficking. The recent cloning of eukaryotic PLD genes from plant, yeast, and human sources has uncovered a novel gene family whose members may be involved in various aspects of signal transduction and membrane traffic.

Phosphatidylserine as a Signal for Recognition and Phagocytosis. Robert A. Schlegel, Pennsylvania State University, Department of Biochemistry and Molecular Biology, University Park, PA 16802 USA.

The amphipathic nature of phospholipids restricts their ability to diffuse transversely from one leaflet of the membrane bilayer to the other. In living cells, movements of this kind are catalyzed by proteins. In the plasma membrane, an ATP-dependent translocase specifically transports phosphatidylserine (PS) from the outer to the inner leaflet of the bilayer, where it is sequestered. Some processes, such as cellular activation and programmed cell death, inactivate the translocase and in coordination activate a nonspecific lipid flipsite, protein in nature, resulting in the appearance of PS on the cell surface. Phosphatidylserine exposed in this fashion is a powerful signal, catalyzing blood coagulation and triggering phagocytosis of apoptotic cells. These mechanisms appear to be common among a variety of cell types, and of ancient evolutionary origin.

Choline and Development of Brain Memory Functions Across the Lifespan. Warren H. Meck, Duke University, Department of Psychology: Experimental, Durham, NC 27708 USA.

One of the most consistant findings in the gerontological literature on cognition is an age–related decline in spatial learning and memory abilities in both rats and humans. These deficits have been noted in tasks that require subjects to locate a place or places to find reward using distal visual environmental cues for accurate navigation. Because the brain areas necessary for proper performance of spatial tasks have been reasonably well characterized in the rat, this animal has been an excellent model in which to test potential therapeutic strategies for ameliorating this cognitive problem. In fact, correlations have been obtained between spatial behavior in mature and aged rats and a number of anatomical, neurochemical, and electrophysiological changes in the hippocampus and frontal cortex. We now report that the beneficial effects of perinatal choline supplementation on memory function shown in young rats (e.g., 2–6 months of age) appear to be permanent. As part of a longitudal study designed to evaluate the longevity of choline-induced memory improvements, male and female Sprague-Dawley rats treated prenatally with choline supplementation (ED 12-17) have been shown to exhibit improved memory performance compared to age-matched control littermates even at 24–30 months of age. For example, aged rats treated prenatally with choline failed to show any age-related decline in choice performance when tested on a 12-arm radial maze with working and reference memory components between the ages of 10 months and 26 months. Between 26–30 months of age these rats were also tested on a retention-interval procedure where a varying delay was inserted between the fourth and fifth correct choice. These delays ranged between 1.25 h and 10 h during which the rat was moved from the maze. After the delay, the rats were replaced on the maze, which was rebaited in the same manner in which they had left it, and were allowed to complete the trial. The data revealed that 30 month old rats given prenatal choline supplementation showed a significantly lower rate of forgetting compared with age-matched controls and were very similar to 2–6 month old rats.

Perinatal Choline Supplementation Alters Neurotrophic Factor– and Transmitter–Specific Septo-Hippocampal Development. Rebekah Loy, University of Rochester, Department of Neurology, 435 E. Henrietta Road, Rochester, NY 14620 USA.

Choline supplementation *in utero* results in a long-lasting facilitation of spatial memory and a variety of correlated brain changes, including decreased choline acetyltransferase (ChAT) activity and increased muscarinic receptor binding in hippocampus and cortex. These early studies suggested that perinatal choline treatment causes an organizational change in cholinergic function, although the nature of the underlying mechanism has been unclear. We have found that the memory improvement correlates with increases in the size of diagonal band neurons immunoreactive for low affinity neurotrophin receptor (p75). Neurons are increased in size in both males and females during development as well as in adult rats, and following choline treatment limited to embryonic days 12–17, as well as following combined pre- and postnatal treatment. In addition, the content of p75 mRNA is increased in the diagonal band, as measured by *in situ* hybridization or RNAse protection assay. However, while NGF protein levels are elevated as much as three-fold in treated hippocampus, there is little or no change in levels of mRNA for the high affinity NGF receptor, TrkA, or in the size of TrkA-immunoreactive diagonal band neurons. Other transmitter-specific changes are also found developmentally in choline-supplemented hippocampus, including a reduction in acetylcholinesterase (AChE) staining in laminae corresponding to septal terminal fields and in interneurons, particularly in temporal denate hilus and CA3. There is also a long-lasting reduction in the staining of hippocampal interneurons immunoreactive for parvalbumin, one marker for GABAergic cells. Thus, choline supplementation elicits transient as well as long-lasting changes in neurotrophins and their receptors as well as changes in the expression of other phenotypic markers characteristic of septohippocampal cholinergic and GABAergic development.

Biochemical Changes in Brains of Animals Exposed to Perinatal Dietary Choline. J.K. Blusztajn, T. Holler, and J.M. Cermak, Boston University School of Medicine, Boston, MA 02118 USA.

Choline is an essential nutrient which serves as a precursor of the neurotransmitter, acetylcholine, in cholinergic neurons, and as a precursor of phosphatidylcholine, sphingomyelin, and plasmenylcholine, phospholipids which collectively are the most abundant components of all biological membranes. We hypothesized that choline availability is important for brain early development. This hypothesis was tested in the offspring of pregnant rats which were fed varying amounts of choline (using choline-deficient, choline-sufficient, and choline-supplemented treatment protocols) during the 11th through 17th day of pregnancy. Others have shown that administration of choline during this period resulted in enhanced performance on memory tests which persisted for life. These behavioral changes were accompanied by neuroanatomical modifications of the brain. Varying the availability of choline during embryonic day (E) 11-E17 affected hippocampal choline acetyltransferase (ChAT), acetylcholinesterase (AChE), and phospholipase D (PLD) activities. On postnatal day (P) 17 and P27, ChAT and AChE activities were highest in rats that had been made prenatally deficient and lowest in the prenatally supplemented male rats. No effect of choline treatment was observed when ChAT and AChE activities were measured on P1, P3, P7, P35, or P90. Thus the postnatal developmental pattern of hippocampal cholinergic markers depends on the availability of choline during embryogenesis. In contrast to the reductions in the activities of ChAT and AChE observed in the hippocampus of rats prenatally supplemented with choline, hippocampal PLD activity was significantly elevated by this treatment (by 30%) on P7 and P21 (but not P1). Moreover, activation of metabotropic glutamate receptors stimulated PLD activity approximately two-fold in all groups. Thus, prenatal choline supplementation stimulates both basal and glutamate-evoked PLD activity in the hippocampus in an age-dependent fashion. The results show that prenatal choline supplementation from E11 to E17, a treatment that leads to a long-lasting improvement in visuospatial memory, also affects biochemical properties of the brain during postnatal development. We conclude that perinatal choline status influences brain development.

Sex Differences in Neural and Behavioral Responses to Perinatal Supplementation with Dietary Choline. Christina L. Williams, Duke University, Department of Psychology: Experimental, Durham, NC 27708 USA.

Cognitive deficits associated with aging and with neurodegenerative diseases such as Alzheimer's disease have been attributed to degeneration of cholinergic neurons in the basal forebrain. Estrogen is known to provide trophic support to cholinergic neurons, and cholinergic neurons in the basal forebrain are known to contain receptors for both estrogen and nerve growth factors. Because males and females differ in their exposure to estrogens, both during the perinatal period of sexual differentiation and during postpuberal life, the cholinergic system develops and functions in a sexually dimorphic hormonal environment. Work from our laboratory has demonstrated that dietary supplementation with choline chloride during both pre- and postnatal development causes long-lasting improvement in memory capacity of male rats of two strains, as assessed using a radial arm maze task as an index of memory function. However, supplemental choline effects on females occur mainly during prenatal development and are of smaller magnitude than the effects in males. This sex difference in the effect of perinatal choline supplementation on memory appears to be dependent upon exposure to steroid hormones during perinatal development. We have found that castration of males at birth, but not at 50 days of age prevents the improvement in memory following perinatal choline supplementation, blocks the increase in hippocampal NGF which is elevated in choline-treated male rats castrated as adults, and prevents the increase in soma size of medial septal neurons immunoreactive for the p75 neurotrophin receptor normally seen in perinatally choline treated adult male rats. These data suggest that there is an interaction between organizational effects of gonadal steroids and organizational effects of supplemental choline on the developing basal forebrain cholinergic system and visuospatial memory.

Origin of Axonal Phosphatidylcholine and Cholesterol in Rat Sympathetic Neurons. Jean E. Vance, Elena Posse de Chaves, Robert B. Campenot, and Dennis E. Vance, University of Alberta, Lipid and Lipoprotein Research Group and Department of Medicine, Biochemistry and Anatomy, and Cell Biology, Edmonton, Alberta, Canada.

Until recently, the paradigm was that all membrane lipids and proteins required for axonal growth were synthesized in cell bodies and transported via anterograde transport into axons. We have used a unique three-compartment model to culture rat sympathetic neurons to show that axons are capable of synthesizing some, but not all, membrane lipids. In this culture system, the cell bodies of rat sympathetic neurons are plated in the center compartment of three-compartmented dishes, and the axons extend into two side compartments containing independent fluid environments. Thus, metabolic events occurring in distal axons alone can be studied. Using this culture system and radiolabeling experiments, we have shown that the major axon membrane phospholipids, including phosphatidylcholine (PC), are synthesized in distal axons. We also demonstrated by direct enzyme assay that enzymes of the CDP-choline pathway for PC synthesis are present in axons. At least 50% of PC of distal axons is made *in situ* in axons. When axons were bathed in a medium devoid of choline, axonal PC synthesis was inhibited and axonal growth was impaired. However, decreased PC synthesis in cell bodies did not inhibit axonal growth. These results suggest that axonal synthesis of PC is required and that synthesis of PC in cell bodies is not the only requirement for normal axonal extension. In contrast to our observation that PC synthesis occurs in distal axons, no synthesis of cholesterol was detected in axons. Inhibition of cholesterol synthesis in cell bodies inhibited axonal growth, but normal growth was restored by the addition of exogenous cholesterol or lipoproteins to axons or cell bodies. Although lipoproteins were able to supply cholesterol for axonal growth, when lipoproteins containing PC were added to either cell bodies or distal axons of choline-deficient neurons (in which axon growth was impaired) normal axon extension did not resume, even though the corresponding concentration of choline in PC of the lipoproteins was 50 times higher than that in normal culture medium. We conclude that the cholesterol required for normal axonal extension can be derived either from cell bodies or from an exogenous supply, whereas the preferred source of PC for axonal growth is *in situ* synthesis in axons.

Platelet Activating Factor Modulated Excitatory Neurotransmitter Release, Gene Expression, and Neuronal Plasticity. Nicolas G. Bazan, Louisiana State University Medical Center School of Medicine, Neuroscience Center, 2020 Gravier Street, Suite B, New Orleans, LA 70112-2234 USA.

The brain's responses to ischemia and seizure initially include membrane depolarization, enhanced accumulation of phospholipase A_2 products such as arachidonic acid and PAF, glutamate release, and influx of calcium ions. The phospholipase A_2 pathway represents a neural inflammatory response by which bioactive lipids become injury signals in repeated seizures (status epilepticus) and ischemia-reperfusion, thus promoting brain damage. The inflammatory mediator PAF is a transcriptional activator of COX-2; BN50730, an intracellular PAF antagonist, blocks this effect. Therefore, we tested the *in vivo* effectiveness of BN50730 in blocking COX-2 induction, and the accumulation of the COX-2 enzyme protein in focal ischemia using the suture model of middle cerebral artery occlusion (MCAO), a model of stroke. Cerebral ischemia and ischemia-reperfusion lead to increased expression and accumulation of COX-2 in the ischemic core as well as in the penumbra in agreement with a recent study. In focal stroke, the penumbra is an important target for drugs that could limit neuronal damage. A single intracerebroventricular injection of BN50730 prevents the MCAO-triggered COX-2 increase. The intracellular PAF antagonist,

BN50730, which blocks this action of PAF has made possible the identification of NFxB, GAS/ISRE, AP-2, and zif-268 as DNA binding activities possibly involved in the induction of COX-2 in hippocampus, because we found that they increase during MCAO and are inhibited by the antagonist. COX-2 accumulation under the above conditions is an event subsequent to the NMDA receptor as its antagonist MK801 inhibits this effect. Thus, brain COX-2 expression may involve the activation by PAF of certain transcription factors, because a PAF antagonist (BN50730) prevents COX-2 induction as well as DNA-binding activities with consensus sequences present in the COX-2 promotor. COX-2, a gene involved in synaptic plasticity responses, may initiate pathological forms of neuroplasticity. Therefore, the PAF/COX-2 pathway is a new drug target in the brain inflammatory response to ischemia.

Importance of Phospholipids in Health and Disease

Lowe Syndrome—A Human Inborn Error of Phosphatidylinositol Metabolism. Sharon F. Suchy, Ann-Marie Leahey, and Robert L. Nussbaum, National Center for Human Genome Research, National Institutes of Health, Building 49, Room 4A 68, Bethesda, MD 20892 USA.

The oculocerebrorenal syndrome of Lowe (OCRL) is a rare X-linked disorder characterized by congenital cataracts, renal tubular dysfunction, and neurological deficits. We and others have demonstrated that OCRL1 encodes a phosphatidylinositol 4,5-bisphosphate 5-phosphatase (Ptdins(4,5)P2 phosphatase) making Lowe syndrome the first identified inherited defect of phosphatidylinositol metabolism in higher eukaryotes. All patient fibroblasts studied to date have reduced or absent ocrl1 protein with reduced Ptdins(4,5)P2 phosphatase activity. The results of immunoprecipitation demonstrate that ocrl1 is the major Ptdins(4,5)P2 phosphatase activity in amniocytes and chorionic villus cells, as it is in fibroblasts, making prenatal diagnosis by biochemical testing feasible. The ocrl1 protein shares six highly conserved motifs with several other known Ptdins(4,5)P2 phosphatases, including INPP5B and synaptojanin. These highly conserved motifs have been proposed to constitute a Ptdins(4,5)P2 phosphatase functional domain. We have identified in one Lowe patient a point mutation that results in an amino acid substitution in one of these highly conserved motifs. The patient has detectable transcript which is indistinguishable from controls in size and amount. We found that fibroblasts from this patient produced ocrl1 protein of normal size, though at reduced levels. However, the Ptdins(4,5)P2 phosphatase activity was 4% of the mean control activity, typical of that observed in other Lowe patients. This case of a point mutation in the putative phosphatidylinositol phosphatase functional domain provides direct evidence that this domain is critical for the phosphatidylinositol phosphatase activity of these proteins. We have also shown that ocrl1 is localized to the Golgi apparatus. Ptdins(4,5)P2 has recently been found to be an activator/essential cofactor for proposed effectors of Golgi membrane trafficking, ARF-GAP, and phospholipase D. Therefore, the regulation of Ptdins(4,5)P2 levels by this 5-phosphatase may be important in the modulation of Golgi vesicular transport. We hypothesize that the primary defect in OCRL is a deficiency of a Golgi Ptdins(4,5)P2 phosphatase which disrupts protein trafficking and in this way precipitates the OCRL phenotype.

Activation of Calcium-Independent Phospholipase A_2 During Hypoxia. Richard W. Gross, Washington University School of Medicine, Division of Bioorganic Chemistry and Molecular Pharmacology, 660 South Euclid Avenue, Campus Box 8020, St. Louis, MO 63110 USA.

The major phospholipase A_2 activity in muscle cells is catalyzed by a calcium-independent, plasmalogen-selective enzyme whose activity is modulated by ATP. To explore the role of this calcium-independent phospholipase A_2 during muscle hypoxia we exploited the specificity inherent in the mechanism–based inhibitor (*E*)-6-(bromomethylene)-3-(1-naphthalenyl)-2-*H*-tetrahydropyran-2-one (BEL) which possesses over a 1,000-fold selectivity for inhibition of calcium-independent versus calcium-dependent phospholipases A_2. These experiments demonstrated that calcium-independent phospholipase A_2 is responsible for the majority of arachidonic acid released in muscle cells during hypoxia. Two mechanisms are envisaged to participate in the accelerated phospholipolysis manifest during hypoxia. First, the release of arachidonic acid catalyzed by the calcium-independent phospholipase A_2 is tightly coupled with glycolytic flux suggesting a fundamental link between phospholipolysis and glycolysis in mammalian cells. Second, nitric axide, released either from sodium nitroprusside or from a thionitroso adduct complexed to albumin, markedly stimulated muscle calcium-independent phospholipase A_2 activity. Collectively, these results demonstrate the importance of calcium-independent phospholipase A_2 in accelerated phospholipolysis during hypoxia and identify two novel mechanisms which can modulate its activity.

Structure and Function of Intracellular PAY Acetyl Hydrolase Isoforms—Miller-Dieker Syndrome—A Human Inborn Error in Platelet-Activating Factor Metabolism. H. Arai, M. Hattori, J. Aoki, and K. Inoue, University of Tokyo, Faculty of Pharmaceutical Science, Hongo, Bunkyo-ku, Tokyo 113, Japan.

The mammalian brain contains several PAF-acetylhydrolase (AH) isoforms in the cytosolic fraction. In the bovine brain, a heterotrimer composed of α, β, and γ-subunits is most abundant, followed by β,γ-dimer and γ,γ-homodimer. As the β,γ-dimer was isolated from the brain, the γ,γ and β,β recombinants exhibited full enzyme activity, indicating that the catalytic site existed on the β and/or γ-subunits. Ser^{47} and Ser^{48} were found to be active serine residues in γ- and β-subunits, respectively. The α-subunit, which is not essential for the catalytic activity *in vitro*, exhibited striking homology (99%) with a protein encoded by the causative gene (*LIS*-1) for Miller-Dieker lissencephaly, a human brain malformation that manifests a smooth cerebral surface and abnormal neural migration. Since the α-subunit was found exclusively in the heterotrimeric complex in the brain. it may play an important regulatory role in PAF metabolism within cells and may affect the migration of neural cells. The expression of the γ-subunit in the developing cerebellum and cerebral cortex is high when neural cell migration is active, and declines as cell migration ceases. The findings support the idea that the enzyme may play an important role in regulation of cell migration during development. α-Subunit contains seven tandem WD-40 repeats and can bind to proteins, such as spectrin which has a PH domain. The overall structure of the present trimeric enzyme resembles that of a heterotrimeric G-protein.

Human Apolipoprotein E: Transgenic Mice Models of Isoform Specific Effects. Donald E. Schmechel and John R. Gilbert, Duke University Medical Center, Department of Medicine (Neurology), Durham VA Medical Center, Durham, NC 27710 USA.

Apolipoprotein E (apoE, protein; APOE, gene) is coded for on human chromosome 19. The three common alleles—2, 3, and 4 differ by only 1-2 amino acid residues, although varying considerably in their binding, biochemical, and functional characteristics. APOE4 allele in single or double dose is considered a risk factor or vulnerability factor for late-onset Alzheimer's Disease (AD). APOE2 confers relative protection and is considered a "longevity" factor in aging studies. I will present the Bryan Alzheimer Research Center's current data on the use of mice strains transgenic for the three specific human APOE genes to model the possible isoform specific effects of apoE on lipid metabolism in brain and related organs. Mice transgenic for the human APOE alleles were created using inbred mice with APOE knockout or null background. Our studies show relative correction of cholesterol status in the transgenic animals compared to the APOE knockouts. In brain tissue, localization of apoE is within neurons similar to the localization of apoE in primate and human brain, but unlike the "normal" rodent localization in glial cells. This permits modeling the possible effects of APOE alleles on neuronal metabolism and possible isoform specific effects on aging and response to brain injury. Some of these effects may influence brain lipid metabolism at both structural and functional levels.

Phosphatidylcholine Is Essential for Normal Secretion of Very Low Density Lipoproteins from Hepatocytes. Dennis E. Vance and Pieter S. Vermeulen, University of Alberta, Lipid and Lipoprotein Research Group and Department of Biochemistry, Edmonton, Alberta, Canada.

Decreased phosphatidylcholine biosynthesis inhibits the secretion of very low density lipoproteins (VLDL) from hepatocytes. There is no apparent effect on the synthesis of the major apolipoprotein associated with VLDL, apo B, nor is apo B translocation into the lumen of the endoplasmic reticulum affected. The nascent particles in the lumen of the endoplasmic reticulum are deficient in phophatidylcholine and the number of VLDL particles in the Golgi fraction is decreased in choline-deficient livers. It is possible that a quality control protease in a post–endoplasmic reticulum compartment degrades apo B on defective particles which are subsequently cleared from the secretory pathway. Recently we investigated whether or not phosphatidylcholine biosynthesis is required for the secretion of carboxyl-truncated apo B 15, 18, 23, 28, and 37 from transfected McArdle RH7777 cells. Transfected cells were choline deprived for one day and then choline supplemented or maintained as choline deficient. Pulse-chase experiments showed that, in the presence of 100 µM choline, the secretion of apo B 28 and 37 was increased by up to 50 and 45%, respectively, whereas the secretion of apo B 15, 18, and 23 was not affected by the addition of choline. Immunoblot analysis also showed that choline in the medium increased the ongoing secretion of apo B 28 and 37 by 30–50%, whereas the secretion of apo B 15, 18, and 23 was unaffected over 24 h. Since only carboxyl-terminal truncations with a size greater than 23% of apo B 100 are able to assemble a neutral lipid core, we conclude that only apo B-truncations that assemble a neutral lipid core require phosphatidylcholine synthesis for secretion from McArdle cells. We also used density fractionation to separate secreted apo B 28 into buoyant and nonbuoyant forms. When choline was added to choline-deficient cells, the secretion of apo B 28 only in the buoyant fraction increased. Since lipoprotein buoyancy is related to the amount of neutral lipid bound, we conclude that the requirement of phosphatidylcholine for apo B secretion is related to the amount of neutral lipid associated with a truncation, rather than the length of apo B.

Requirements for Dietary Choline During Pregnancy. Steven H. Zeisel and Mei-Heng Mar, University of North Carolina, Department of Nutrition, CB #7400, McGavran-Greenberg, Chapel Hill, NC 27599-7400 USA.

Choline is an important nutrient which is actively transported from mother to fetus across the placenta, and from mother to infant across the mammary gland. Thus, pregnancy and lactation are times when dietary requirements for choline may be increased. Pregnant rats eating AIN-76A diet (with and without choline) for six days (days 12–18 gestation) were compared to nonmated female and male rats eating the same diet. Similarly, lactating rats were compared to nonmated female rats, both groups eating these same diets for 25 days (gestation day 12–postpartum day 15). We measured choline and choline metabolites in livers on the last day of feeding. Nonmated female rats, eating the control diet, had higher hepatic choline metabolite concentrations than did male rats (choline, 98%; betaine, 96%; and phosphorylcholine, 55% higher), pregnant rats (phosphorylcholine, 47%; and betaine, 42% higher) or lactating rats (phosphorylcholine, 49%; phosphatidylcholine, 37%, and betaine, 273% higher). We found that nonmated females eating a choline-deficient diet had only a modest diminution of the labile choline metabolite PCho in liver, compared with similar rats eating a control diet (33% decrease). When compared to similar rats fed a choline-adequate diet, pregnant rats had significantly greater diminution of hepatic phosphorylcholine (83% decrease) when fed a choline-deficient diet than did nonmated females. Lactating rats were the most sensitive to choline deficiency, with liver phosphorylcholine decreasing 88% (compared to similar rats on control diet; we observed a 12% decrease compared to controls in nonmated females fed the deficient diet for the same 25-day period). Our data suggest that the nonpurified diet offered in the laboratory does not provide sufficient choline to meet the extraordinary demands of pregnancy and lactation. The intake of extra dietary choline may be advantageous during pregnancy and lactation in rats. Choline is also important for normal brain development—there are two sensitive periods in development of rat brain during which treatment with choline results in long–lasting facilitation of spatial memory. The first occurs during embryonic days 12–17 and another during postnatal days 16–30. These two sensitive periods correlate with neurogenesis of cholinergic cells (prenatal) and with synaptogenesis (postnatal). Choline supplementation during these critical periods elicits a constant percentage improvement in choice performance at all stages of training for a visuospatial task (12-arm radial maze). Thus, our studies on choline requirements during pregnancy may be important with respect to understanding brain and neural tube development.

Homocysteine and Vascular Disease: Role for Folate, Choline, and Lipoprotein in Homocysteine Metabolism. Kilmer S. McCully, Veterans Administration Medical Center, 830 Chalkstone Avenue, Providence, RI 02908 USA.

The atherogenic effect of homocysteine was discovered by analysis of the pathology of genetic disorders of homocysteine metabolism. Homocysteine causes arteriosclerotic placques in experimental animals, and epidemiological studies have established hyperhomocysteinemia as a major risk factor for human arteriosclerosis. Homocysteine synthesis is controlled in liver by the inhibitory effects of adenosylmethionine on methylenetetrahydrofolate reductase and by stimulation of cystathionine synthesis. The reactive anhydride, homocysteine thiolactone, is synthesized in liver from methionine, and catalyzed by methionyl tRNA synthase, where it is associated with membrane lipids. Folate deficiency causes elevated blood homocysteine because of reduced formation of methyltetrahydrofolate and decreased transfer of methyl groups to methyl cobalamin and homocysteine to synthesize methionine. Betaine, derived from choline by oxidation, transfers a methyl group to homocysteine to form methionine by an alternate transmethylation pathway only in liver. Betaine is partially effective in lowering blood homocysteine in homocystenuria and in renal failure. The atherogenic effect of homocysteine thiolactone is mediated by the aggregation of low-density lipoprotein through helix coil transitions and causes interaction with cultured macrophages via phagocytosis and receptor uptake, thus forming foam cells. Cell culture proteoglycans that are deficient in cystathionine synthase are converted from fibrillar to aggregated conformation, associated with increased sulfate binding and increased formation of phosphoadenosine phosphosulfate from homocysteine. Malignant cells synthesize increased homocysteine thiolactone because of a thioretinaco deficiency, resulting in the homocysteinylation of proteins, aggregation of nucleoproteins, and membrane simplification. Thioretinaco ozonide forms an active-site disulfonium complex that binds ATP of F_1F_0 complexes of mitochondrial membranes, coupling reduction of bound oxygen, electron transport, and proton pumping through mitochondrial membranes. Loss of thioretinaco ozonide causes increased accumulation of oxygen radicals within cells, promoting oxidative modification of low-density lipoprotein, endothelial injury, platelet aggregation, thrombosis, and other features of developing arteriosclerotic plaques.

Poster Presentations

Conversion of Dihydroceramide to Ceramide: Involvement of a Desaturase. L. Geeraert, G.P. Mannaerts, and P.P. Van Veldhoven, Katholieke Universiteit Leuven, Campus Gasthuisberg, Afd Farmacologie, Herestraat 49, B-3000 Leuven, Belgium.

The 4-*trans* double bond, present in the sphingoid base moiety of most sphingolipids, is thought to be introduced during the biosynthesis of these lipids at the level of dihydroceramide (*N*-acyl-sphinganine). The produced ceramide (*N*-acyl-sphingenine) serves as the precursor for sphingomyelin and glycosphingolipids. The enzyme(s) responsible for the double bond formation is poorly characterized. In order to study this enzymic activity, the production of water in rat (permeabilized) hepatocytes or rat liver homogenates, incubated with a truncated dihydroceramide analog, *N*-hexanoyl-[4,5-^{3}H]-sphinganine (in a 1:1 molar complex with BSA), was followed. Compared to intact cells (activity = 7.42 $\pm$ 0.66 nmol/min per 10^8 cells), the formation of ceramide was severely decreased in permeabilized cells (0.51 ± 0.10 nmol/min per 10^8 cells). The addition of various known cofactors for oxidases and dehydrogenases to permeabilized cells was not able to restore the activity, but NADPH and ATP appeared to stimulate activity. The NADPH effect was the first hint that a desaturase might be involved, while the ATP effect could reflect the requirement for cellular transport. Compounds that interact with various parts of known desaturase systems (artificial electron acceptors, such as methylene blue, Janus green, menadione, and DCPIP; NEM, an inactivator of flavoproteins; and CN^-, a very potent inhibitor of stearyl-CoA desaturase) were strong inhibitors of dihydroceramide desaturation, not only in intact hepatocytes, but also in permeabilized hepatocytes (fortified with NADPH/ATP) and in rat liver homogenates (under optimized assay conditions). In summary, our data clearly point to the involvement of a desaturase system that appeared to reside in the endoplasmic reticulum in the conversion of dihydroceramide to ceramide.

Quantification of Phosphatidylethanol in Human Blood. Torsten Gunnarsson and Anders Å. Karlsson, Lund University, Chemical Ecology and Ecotoxicology, S-223 62 Lund, Sweden; Per Hansson and Christer Alling, University Hospital, Department of Medical Neurochemistry, Institute of Laboratory Medicine, S-221 85 Lund, Sweden; and Goran Odham, Stockholm University, Laboratory for Analytical Environmental Chemistry, S-106 92 Stockholm, Sweden.

High-performance liquid chromatography with evaporative light scattering detection (ELSD) or electrospray mass spectrometry was used to determine the concentration of phosphatidylethanol (Peth) in extracts of human blood samples. Peth is a "pathological" phospholipid formed by the action of phospholipase D in the presence of ethanol. Separation was performed using a Lichrospher 100 DIOL column packed at 950 bar and a normal phase, multisolvent binary gradient system, consisting of hexane, *n*-propanol, water, acetic acid, and triethylamine. In a human blood sample, the limit of detection with ELSD was about 200 pmol ($\approx$125 ng) of the injected compound. Peth was found in whole blood and in red blood cells (RBC) but could not be detected in plasma. Decreasing concentrations of Peth, from about 15 nmol/mL blood, could be followed in alcohol addicts more than 20 days after the beginning of an alcohol-free period. The rate of Peth decrease differed between blood and RBC as well as between different patients. The molecular species of Peth contained mainly combinations of 16:0, 18:1, and 18:2 O-acylated fatty acids. These combinations are also common among the other phospholipid classes in the sample.

Sphingomyelins in Bovine Milk—Determination of Molecular Species Composition Using Liquid Chromatography–Mass Spectrometry with Atmospheric Pressure Chemical Ionization (APCI) and Electrospray Ionization (ES). Anders Å. Karlsson, Lund University, Chemical Ecology and Ecotoxicology, Ecology Building, S-223 62 Lund, Sweden.

A sphingomyelin fraction of polar lipids from bovine milk (whey) has been analyzed with straight-phase high-performance liquid chromatography–mass spectrometry (MS). Either atmospheric pressure chemical ionization (APCI) or electrospray ionization (ES) was used. Ions characteristic of the long-chain bases (LCB) and the

N-ecylated fatty acids (FA) were formed by positive ionization APCI-MS/MS. The cleavage pattern and ions produced using APCI were comparable with those previously obtained with discharge-assisted thermospray (plasmaspray) ionization. Major molecular species were composed of monounsaturated LCB with 16 (*d*-16:1) or 18 (*d*-18:1) carbon atoms together with saturated *N*-acylated FA with 16, 22, 23, or 24 carbon atoms in the chain. In addition, *d*-17:1- and *d*-19:1-LCB were present in addition to small amounts of the saturated LCB *d*-16:0, *d*-17:0, and *d*-18:0. The molecular species composition of the sphingomyelin fraction will be presented. Mass spectra of molecular species LCS and *N*-acylated FA, together with data on combinations of LCB/FA present in the sample will also be included.

Determination of Phospholipids Using Straight-Phase Liquid Chromatography–Electrospray Mass Spectrometry. Anders Å. Karlsson, Lund University, Chemical Ecology and Ecotoxicology, Ecology Building, S-223 62 Lund, Sweden.

Straight-phase liquid chromatography (LC)–electrospray (ES) mass spectrometry was used for the separation and detection of all major phospholipids, such as phosphatidic acid (PA), phosphatidylglycerol (PG), phosphatidylethanolamine (PE), phosphatidylcholine (PC), phosphatidylserine (PS), phosphatidylinositol (PI), and sphingomyelin. The detection limit was approximately 5 pg (~ 7 fmol) phospholipid/μL injected solvent in multiple reaction monitoring (MRM) mode with ES negative ionization. Statistical data on dose–response variation, as well as results from analyses of biological samples will be presented. Problems connected with analysis at, and slightly above the detection limit will be discussed. The analyses have been performed overnight and up to 50 hours. The automation setup will also be described.

Phospholipid Molecular Species Composition of Developing Fetal Guinea Pig Brain. Graham C. Burdge and Anthony D. Postle, Child Health, University of Southampton, UK.

We have investigated the effect of increasing gestational age upon fetal guinea pig brain phosphatidylcholine (PC) and phosphatidylethanolamine (PE) molecular species composition. PC and PE were purified from fetal brains (n = 6/time point), and the molecular species were resolved by HPLC with postcolumn fluorescence detection. Brain PC contained predominately PC16:0/16:0 and PC16:0/18:1, while PE was composed mainly of polyunsaturated species. Increasing gestational age between day 25 and term (day 68) was accompanied by minor changes in PC composition, but was associated with marked differential changes in PE species content. For example, 22:6ω-3 was accumulated primarily into *sn*-1 16:0 and 18:1ω-9 species between day 25 and 35, and into *sn*-1 18:0 species from day 35 to term. These results show that the maturation of the fetal brain is accompanied by programmed changes in the membrane phospholipid composition, which suggests individual molecular species may have specific functions at defined stages in development.

Metabolic Strategies for Altered Hepatic Phosphatidylcholine Composition in the Pregnant Rat and Guinea Pig. Graham C. Burdge, and Anthony D. Postle, Child Health, University of Southampton, UK.

Hepatic and plasma PC16:0/22:6 content is increased in the pregnant rat and guinea pig, which may facilitate 22:6ω-3 supply to the developing brain. Mechanisms for hepatic phosphatidylcholine (PC) biosynthesis were investigated in the pregnant rat and guinea pig. CDP:[^{14}C]choline and CDP:[^{14}C]ethanolamine incorporation into microsomal phospholipids *in vitro* indicated substantial modification to the composition of specific diacylglycerol (DAG) substrate pools in pregnancy. In the pregnant rat, the 16:0/22:6 content was increased in DAG pools incorporated into PC and phosphatidylethanolamine (PE). In contrast, only DAG destined for PE synthesis showed an increased 16:0/22:6 content in the guinea pig. [^{14}C]choline and [^{14}C]methionine incorporations into PC *in vivo* showed increased *de novo* synthesis in the pregnant rat, while PE *N*-methylation was elevated in the guinea pig. The specificity of acyl remodeling was not altered in either animal species. These results suggest that the rat and guinea pig have evolved markedly different strategies for increased hepatic PC16:0/22:6 content in pregnancy and indicate PC16:0/22:6 may play a unique role in 22:6ω-3 metabolism.

Antineoplastic Activity of Alkylphosphocholines and Alkylphosphocholine Liposomes: A Review of Recent Knowledge. D. Arndt, I. Fichtner, and R. Zeisig, Max Delbrück Center for Molecular Medicine, D-13122 Berlin, Germany.

The similarity of liposomes to cell membranes and their ability to carry substances forms the basis of their scientific and industrial applications. Liposomes are generated normally from inert phosphoglycerolipids containing two hydrophobic fatty acid chains, for example phosphatidylcholine. Phospholipid vesicles have proven to be a valuable carrier for drugs, genetic material, or cosmetics. Our approach in the field of experimental cancer therapy applies a lipid with antitumor properties as the primary constituent for liposome formation. Such lipids are alkylphosphocholines (APC). Alkylphosphocholines represent a new class of non-DNA-interactive compounds for experimental and clinical cancer therapy. Alkylphosphocholines are substances with a wide spectrum of biological properties, such as cytotoxity against tumor cells *in vitro* and *in vivo*, modulation of phospholipid metabolism, induction of differentiation in malignant cells, activation of cytotoxic macrophages, inhibition of neoplastic cell invasion in normal tissues, and interference with different steps of signaling pathways. Liposome formation is possible with alkylphosphocholines (C_{12}–C_{20}) as the main lipid constituent, if cholesterol and small amounts of a charged lipid are present. The behavior and the potential of these alkylphosphocholine liposomes in the field of experimental cancer research will be discussed. APC and APC liposomes show remarkable activity against some human mammary carcinomas in nude mice, while other tumors are unaffected. The indirect action is characterized by the enhancement of cytotoxic properties of macrophages [increased production of NO radicals and increased release of tumor necrosis factor (TNF)]. The major side effects of the APCs, especially gastrointestinal toxicity and hemolysis, were reduced by the use of the liposomal preparations. Like conventional liposomes, APC liposomes are usually rapidly cleared from circulation by the mononuclear phagocyte system (MPS). The uptake of APC liposomes by the MPS can be significantly inhibited by the incorporation of polyethylendeglycol-linked lipids into the bilayer.

Didecanoylphosphatidylcholine Is a Superior Substrate for Assaying Mammalian Phospholipase D. Anne M. Vinggaard, Torben Jensen, and Harald S. Hansen, Department of Biological Sciences, The Royal Danish School of Pharmacy, Copenhagen, Denmark; and Clive P. Morgan and Shamshad Cockcroft, University College London, Department of Physiology, London WC1E 6JJ, UK.

Phospholipase D (PLD) activity in crude or solubilized membranes from mammalian tissues is difficult to detect with the current assay techniques, unless a high concentration of radio nuclides is present in the substrate and/or long incubation times are employed. Furthermore, PLD activity from cultured cells can only be detected by the available assay techniques, when GTPγS and a cytosolic factor (usually Arf) is added. In this paper, we report that a short-chained phosphatidylcholine, *i.e.* [^{3}H]didecanoylphosphatidylcholine (C_{10}-PC), is superior as an exogenous substrate for assaying mammalian PLD activity both in cells and tissues. C_{10}-PC was compared to [^{3}H]dipalmitoylphosphatidylcholine (C_{16}-PC) as a substrate for PLD activities from membranes of human neutrophils, human placenta, and porcine brain or from placental cytosol. C_{10}-PC was superior to C_{16}-PC by a factor of 2–28 depending on the assay conditions and tissue, and it allowed the detection of Arf-sensitive PLD activity without addition of PIP_2 and Arf. Thus, the inclusion of DDPC in future assays will be of great value in further work on purifying and determining the regulation and function of this enzyme.

Glutamate-Induced Formation of *N*-acyl-phosphatidylethanolamine (NAPE) and *N*-acylethanolamine (NAE) in Cortical Neurons. Harald S. Hansen, L. Lauritzen, A.M. Strand, A.M. Vinggaard, A. Schousboe, and A. Frandsen. Department of Biological Science, The Royal Danish School of Pharmacy, Copenhagen, DK-2100, Denmark.

We have shown that NAPE and NAE accumulated in rat cortical neurons in response to cell culture maturation, calcium ionophore, and the neurotoxic neurotransmitter glutamate (1). In neurons cultured for 6 days, glutamate-induced NAPE and NAE formation dose dependently and linearly for 0–150 min. NAPE formation in immature neurons (2 days in culture, at a developmental stage in which glutamate is not toxic) could not be induced by 100 μM glutamate, whereas A23187 induced a small formation. The glutamate-induced NAPE formation in 6-day-old neurons could be prevented by a calcium-deficient medium, and by the NMDA-receptor antagonist TCP but not the AMPA/kainate-receptor antagonist CNQX, indicating the involvement of the NMDA-receptor. Other toxic stimuli, such as changing to fresh serum-containing medium or the addition of 5 mM NaN_3 stimulated NAPE formation. No formation of NAPE could be detected in rat Leydig cells, astrocytes, cardiomyocytes, or in human fibroblast and apoptotic leukemia cells. Thus, glutamate-induced NAPE and NAE formation is calcium-dependent and mediated via the NMDA-receptor. It seems to be associated with glutamate-induced neuronal death which occurred at a slower time scale. We speculate that the formation of NAPE and NAE, including *N*-arachidonoyl-ethanolamine (anandamide), is an early sign of neuronal toxicity.

Separation and Quantification of Polyphosphoinositides Using Normal-Phase HPLC and Evaporative Light-Scattering Detection or Electrospray Mass

Spectrometry. Torsten Gunnarsson and Anders Karlsson, Lund University, Chemical Ecology and Ecotoxicology, S-223 62 Lund, Sweden; Bengt Jergil, Lund University, Biochemistry, Centre for Chemistry, S-221 00 Lund, Sweden; Peter Michelsen, Nycomed Innovation, IDEON-Malmö, S-205 12 Malmö, Sweden; and Goran Odham, Stockholm University, Laboratory for Analytical Environmental Chemistry, S-106 92 Stockholm, Sweden.

Baseline separation of polyphosphoinositides [PIP] (phosphatidylinositol monophosphate [PIP] and phosphatidylmositol diphosphate [PIP_2]) was performed within 17 min. on a Spherisorb silica (5 µM) column (10 cm × 2 mm i.d.) packed at 950 bar. The analyses were performed using a multisolvent binary gradient system consisting of chloroform, methanol, water, and ammonia. The detection limit of PIP with evaporative light-scattering detection was about 300 ng of injected compound. Good separation was also achieved between some of the glycero-phospholipid classes. Phosphatidic acid, phosphatidylcholine, and phosphatidylserine eluted as single peaks, whereas phosphatidylglycerol, phosphatidylethanolamine, and phosphatidylinositol eluted together. The method has been applicated on natural membrane samples with electrospray mass spectrometry for molecular species evaluation.

Gastric Mucosa Protection by Phosphatidylcholine (PC). Armin Wendel, Nattermann Phospholipid GmbH, Nattermannallee 1, D-50829 Cologne, Germany.

The effect of co-administration of exogenous PC on the oral gastrotoxicity of various nonsteroidal anti-inflammatory drugs (NSAID) was studied in rats that received a three-day bread diet followed by 24 h fasting. Gastric mucosal lesions were measured 3.5 h after oral administration of the drug or drug/PC mixtures. PC reduced the ulcer index by the maximum of 82% for aspirin, 47% for indometacin, 78% for phenylbutazone, 94% for diclofenac, 78% for piroxicam, and 53% for sudoxicam. In a follow-up human study on 20 subjects with gastric pain, the oral treatment with PC from soybean after three days relieved pain in 15 and improved 3 patients.

CTP:Cholinephosphate Cytidylyltransferase (CT) Is Redistributed to the Perinuclear Cytoskeleton in Differentiating IMR-32 Neuroblastoma Cells. Alan N. Hunt and Anthony D. Postle, Child Health, University of Southampton, UK.

Increased flux through the *de novo* pathway of cellular phosphatidylcholine biosynthesis is usually accompanied by redistribution of CT from soluble to particulate fractions. Indirect immunofluorescence of IMR-32 human neuroblastoma cells in cycle, using polyclonal anti-CT directed to either the N-terminal sequence or whole recombinant CT, showed both diffuse cytoplasmic and nuclear staining. An intense nuclear translocation of CT was seen within 8 h of commitment to differentiation by addition of retinoic acid, concomitant with a rearrangement of the actin cytoskeleton visualized with rhodamine-phalloidin. Laser-scanning confocal microscopy revealed that this CT was largely perinuclear and colocalized with an F-actin net, offering intriguing regulatory possibilities.

The Importance of Phospholipids in Health and Disease. Leonard S. Girsh, Immunopath Profile, Inc., 825 Warfield Lane, Huntington Valley, PA 19006.

The significance of phospholipids in the pathogenesis of the immunological and allergic diseases, including asthma, and in the therapeutics and the principles of management of immunologic and allergic diseases, including asthma, are investigated.

Sphingomyelin Digestion in the Rat Intestinal Tract. Lena Nyberg, Swedish Dairies' Association, S-223 70 Lund, Sweden; Åke Nilsson and Pia Lundgren, Department of Medicine, University Hospital of Lund, S-221 85, Lund, Sweden; and Rui-Dong Duan, Department of Cell Biology 1, University Hospital of Lund, S-221 85, Lund, Sweden.

The extension and capacity of sphingomyelin (SM) digestion *in vivo* was examined. After feeding rats 0.2, 6.6, or 32 µmoles ^{3}H-sphingosine-labeled milk SM (^{3}H-SM), radioactivity was measured in intestinal contents and tissues 2, 4, and 8 h later. The amount of radioactivity in the contents of small intestine increased with the dose of ^{3}H-SM; 9% of given dose with 0.2 µmoles, 34% with 6.6 µmoles, and 71% with 32 µmoles, respectively, after 2 h. The lowest tissue radioactivity was found in duodenum and proximal jejunum, while the highest was in the distal jejunum and proximal ileum. Ceramide contained 3–21% of radioactivity in the intestinal tissue; the proportion varied with the dose given, region of the intestine, and time after administration. After administration of 6.6 or 32 µmoles SM, significant amounts of intact SM and ceramide were found in intestinal contents, colon, and excreted feces. The colon was exposed to ceramide in an amount that was proportional to the dose of SM fed. SM digestion is thus a process extending over the whole intestine and occurs mainly in the middle and lower parts of the small intestine. The site of digestion coincides with the distribution of the alkaline SMase, which we had identified previously, indicating that this enzyme catalyzes the first step in digestion. The extension and limited capacity of SM digestion leads to an exposure of the lower small intestine and colon to SM and sphingolipid metabolites, known to be important lipid messengers that regulate cell proliferation, differentiation, and apoptosis.

Phospholipid-Mediated Oxidation of LDL. Phillip Greenspan and Pingping Lou, University of Georgia, College of Pharmacy, Athens, GA 30602-2356 USA.

The oxidation of low-density lipoprotein (LDL) is thought to be an important process in atherogenesis. While previous *in vitro* studies have focused exclusively on the oxidation of LDL in the absence of exogenously added lipids, phospholipids found in the atheroma should also be subject to oxidation and participate in the LDL modification process. To examine the relationship between the phospholipid oxidation and the subsequent modification of LDL, we incubated 250 µM egg phosphatidylcholine (PC) with 10 µM ferrous sulfate and 50 µM ascorbic acid in 10 mM Tris, pH 7.0. After 18 h at 37°C, lipoperoxidation of egg PC was ascertained by the formation of significant amounts of TBARS. The addition of LDL (100 µg protein/mL) to this solution elevated the TBARS and increased the electrophoretic mobility of the lipoprotein. LDL, incubated with iron and ascorbate in the absence of PC, or LDL treated with iron and ascorbate in the presence of a synthetic PC containing saturated acyl chains, did not become modified. LDL that was incubated with egg PC, iron, and ascorbate was metabolized by macrophages to a far greater extent than native LDL or LDL treated with PC alone. Probucol (10 µM), an antioxidant, inhibited the modification of LDL. These results demonstrate that the oxidation of PC can mediate the modification of LDL.

Lowering Serum Cholesterol by Topical Treatment with Soy Phosphatidyl-choline. S.L. Hsia, Jin Lin He, Mitchell Mandel, and Catherine W. Froelich, University of Miami School of Medicine, Miami, FL 33136 USA; and Xiao Ming Xu, Henan Electric Power Hospital, Zheng Zhou, China.

We previously observed the hypocholesterolemic and antiatherogenic effects of topically applied soy phosphatidylcholine (PC) in rabbits with heritable hypercholes-terolemia. In a further study, 14 normolipidemic men volunteered to take topical PC. They received topical PC (1.4 g) in a liposomal form, once daily for 30 days. At the end of the study, their mean serum cholesterol decreased 10%, without elevation of circulating liver enzymes. In another study, 16 hypercholesterolemic men and 20 hypercholerolemic women (serum cholesterol above 230 mg/dL) were treated with topical PC (6.6 g) in an alcoholic solution, twice weekly for 8 weeks. Their serum cholesterol decreased 25% and LDL cholesterol decreased 23%, without undesirable side effects. There was also a noticeable, although not statistically significant, decrease of serum triglycerides. We propose that topical PC may be therapeutically useful for the treatment of hypercholesterolemia and warrants further clinical studies.

Fundamental Studies of Structure–Activity Relationships in Antineoplastic Lipid and Phospholipid Analogs. George S. Attard and Wendy S. Smith, University of Southampton, Department of Chemistry, 50 University Road, Highfield Southampton SO17 1BJ, UK.

A systematic investigation has been conducted into the relationship between chem-ical structure and *in vitro* activity of a wide range of antineoplastic lipid and phospho-lipid analogs. The data from these studies reveal a striking correlation between the EC_{50} and the critical micellar concentration (cmc) of the compounds. In general, the EC_{50} is at least an order of magnitude lower than the cmc, confirming that cytostasis is not a consequence of a detergent effect. The principal factor affecting activity was found to be the effective cross-section of the hydrophilic headgroups rather than their chemical nature. This supports earlier suggestions that the mode of action of these compounds is unlikely to involve specific interactions with cellular proteins. These observations have led to simple rules for the design of compounds with enhanced activity and may pro-vide important insights into the mode of action of phospholipid analogs.

Absorption and Metabolism of the Absorption Enhancer Didecanoylphos-phatidylcholine in Rabbit Nasal Epithelium *In Vivo*. Charlotte Vermehren, The Royal Danish School of Pharmacy, Department of Pharmacy, Copenhagen, Denmark; Peter B. Johansen, Novo Nordisk A/S, Growth Hormone Biology, Niels Steensensvej 8, Gentofte, Denmark; and Harald S. Hansen, The Royal Danish School of Pharmacy, Department of Biology, Copenhagan, Denmark.

The absorption enhancer, didecanoylphosphatidylcholine (DDPC), can improve the nasal absorption of human growth hormone in rabbits. We elucidated the uptake in the tissue and metabolism of 1,2-di[1-^{14}C]-decanoyl1L-3-phosphatidylcholine and 1,2-didecanoyl-L-3-phosphatidyl-[*N*-methyl-^{3}H]choline in rabbit nasal mucosas *in vivo*. One minute after nasal application of DDPC, 0.5–0.7% of the applied dose was absorbed in the mucosa. The retained radoactivity left the tissue in less than 2 h. At $t = 1$ min. only 0.1% of the applied dose was found as intact DDPC in the nasal mucosa. The other labeled lipophilic compounds were decanoic acid, phosphatidylcholine, neutral lipid, and small amounts of lysoDDPC and phosphatidylethanolamine (PE). Analysis of water-soluble metabolites revealed formation of phosphorylcholine, glycerophosphorylcholine, cytidindiphosphatecholine (CDP-choline), and slight amounts of choline. Detection of these metabolites suggests that DDPC was rapidly cleared from the mucosa, partly by degradation by phospholipases. In addition, DDPC metabolites were reutilized in the formation of CDP-CHO and PE together with DDPC being reacylated with endogenous fatty acids. Thus, the very rapid catabolism of DDPC with the formation of mainly decanoic acid raises the question whether some of the absorption enhancing properties attributed to DDPC may be mediated by decanoic acid.

N-Terminal Mutants of Human Secreted Phospholipase A$_2$. David C. Wilton, University of Southampton, Department of Biochemistry, Bassett Crescent East, Southampton SO16 7PX, UK.

Human nonpancreatic secreted phospholipse A$_2$ (hnpsPLA$_2$) is of considerable interest because of its involvement in a number of inflammatory disorders. For example, elevated levels of the enzyme are found in the appropriate extracellular fluid in septic shock, rheumatoid arthritis, and asthma. The precise function of this enzyme and its role in the inflammation process is not clear. More information is required about the structure/function of this enzyme and, in particular, the interfacial and heparin-binding properties of the enzyme. This approach will be facilitated by site-directed mutagenesis. A gene coding for this enzyme has been synthesized and overexpressed in *E. coli* and the system will be described. The enzyme expressed has been mutated to provide an *N*-terminal alanine (N1A) and this allows the initiator methionine to be removed by the *E. coli* aminopeptidase. Further mutations have been produced including a tryptophan-containing mutant, N1A, V3W; the properties of this mutant will be described.

Influence of the Nature of the Fatty Acids Esterified in Phosphatidylcholine from HDL on Lymphocyte Proliferation. F. Thies and P.C. Calder, Department of Biochemistry, South Parks Road, Oxford OX1 3QU, UK.

In vitro studies have shown that polyunsaturated fatty acids (PUFA) inhibit lymphocyte activities, such as proliferation, IL 2 production, cytotoxicity, natural killer cell activity, and antigen presentation. Furthermore, PUFA-rich diets have been shown to be able to have beneficial effects in some types of inflammatory and autoimmune diseases. Fatty acids (FA) from the diet are redistributed in the plasma in different forms. Among these are the high-density lipoproteins (HDL), which are able to provide some growth factors, perhaps FA esterified to phospholipids (PL), necessary for lymphocyte proliferation. Phosphatidylcholine (PC) is the main PL present in HDL. It is possible that the FA composition of PC in HDL can modulate lymphocyte activities. Therefore, we investigated the influence of HDL enriched with different PC (PC-16:0/18:1, 18:0/18:2, and 16:0/20:4) on lymphocyte proliferation in comparison with control HDL. Freshly purified control and PC-enriched HDL (10–200 µg protein-equivalent HDL) were incubated for 48 h with human lymphocytes (2×10^6 cells/mL) using different culture media (without or containing human normal or delipoproteinized serum) in the presence of a mitogen (Concanavalin A). We found that HDL inhibit lymphocyte proliferation in a dose-dependent manner whatever the culture medium used. Moreover, HDL enriched with PUFA-containing PC, especially PC-18:2, were more inhibitory than the control HDL. We conclude that the composition of the FA esterified to the PL of HDL could significantly affect lymphocyte function.

Quantitative Determination of Phospholipids: Validation of the ^{31}P-NMR-Method. Bernd W.-K. Diehl, Werner Ockels, Helmut Herling, Ricarda Unger, Stephanie Winkler, Spectral Service GmbH, Vogelsanger Str. 250, D-50825 Köln, Germany.

The study shows the validity of the quantitative determination of egg-phospholipids in a pharmaceutical liposome preparation using the ^{31}P-NMR-method. Subjects of validation were instrument precision, method precision, selectivity, recovery, robustness of the method including variation of pH-value, variation of the ternary solvent mixture, variation of the number of scans, amount of sample (ratio sample/standard), time between sample preparation and measurement, and data evaluation. Method precision (reproducibility) and instrument precision show for main components a standard deviation <1%, components near the limit of quantitation have a standard deviation below 5%. For the liposome lyophilisate preparation the extraction recovery of the phospholipids is 100%. The analysis method is robust. It is almost insensitive to variation in sample preparation and parameters of measurement. Prepared samples can be stored up to 5 days at room temperature (typical <24 h) until they are measured without negative influence of the results.

Chapter 1

Sphingomyelin and Other Sphingomyelin Metabolites in Cell Signaling and Disease

Eva-Maria Schmelz, Mariana Nikolova-Karakashian, Elaine Wang, and Alfred H. Merrill, Jr.

Emory University School of Medicine, Atlanta, GA

Sphingomyelin

Sphingomyelin (N-acyl sphingosine-1-phosphocholine or ceramide phosphocholine) (Fig. 1.1) is found in all tissues and lipoproteins, where it is located primarily in the plasma membrane and associated compartments (e.g., endocytic vesicles and lysosomes) (1,13). The sphingomyelin molecule is composed of (1) a long-chain (sphingoid) base, of which sphingosine (*trans-4*-sphingenine) is the major species, but lesser amounts of sphinganines, 4-hydroxysphinganines, and homologs having varying chain lengths are also found; (2) an amide-linked fatty acid, which is typically saturated and with a chain length of 16 to 24 carbon atoms (unbranched); and (3) a phosphorylcholine headgroup. Although sphingomyelin is generally thought to be the only phosphosphingolipid of mammals, small amounts of ceramide phosphorylethanolamine have been seen in liver tissue, and additional phosphosphingolipids are common in other organisms.

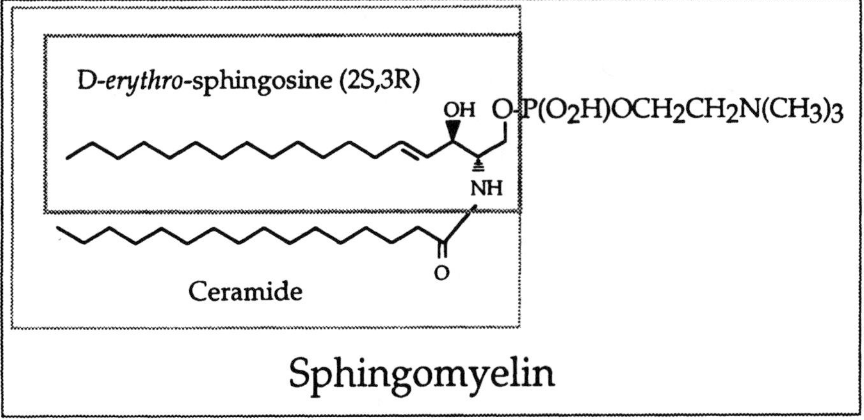

Fig. 1.1. Structure of sphingomyelin with the sphingosine and ceramide moieties delineated.

Sphingomyelin and Cell Signaling

Sphingomyelin has long been known to be hydrolyzed to ceramide, which is further cleaved to sphingosine and phosphorylated to sphingosine 1-phosphate, as shown in Fig. 1.2. Although sphingomyelin turnover was initially studied from the perspective of the diseases that involve genetic defects in sphingomyelin turnover (e.g., Niemann-Pick's disease), the field has shifted to explore the role of these metabolites (as well as ceramide 1-phosphate and sphingosylphosphorylcholine) as a new category of "lipid second messenger," because they are potent modulators of cell growth, differentiation, diverse cell behaviors, and programmed cell death (2).

The current paradigm (Fig. 1.2) is that cytokines induce the activation of sphingomyelinase(s) and the turnover of sphingomyelin to ceramide, which activate protein phosphatases and kinases (8,9); growth factors, on the other hand, stimulate sphingomyelinase(s), ceramidase(s) and sphingosine kinase(s), leading to the formation of sphingosine 1-phosphate, a potent mitogen that triggers release of intracellular calcium (6,18). One might suspect that cellular responses to some agents could involve more than one sphingolipid "second messenger," as is found in other lipid signaling pathways. We have made a number of observations that indicate that such is the case for the response of rat hepatocytes to IL-1β, as will be described in the next section.

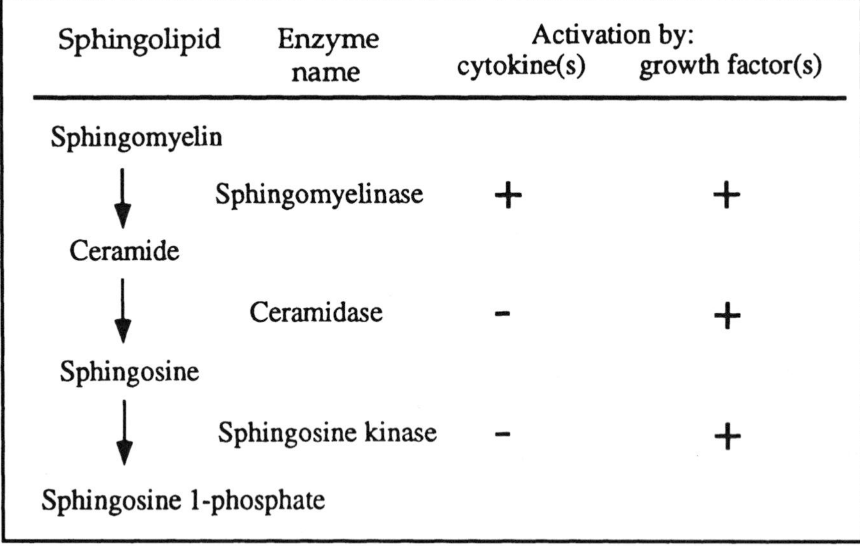

Sphingolipid	Enzyme name	Activation by: cytokine(s)	growth factor(s)
Sphingomyelin			
↓	Sphingomyelinase	+	+
Ceramide			
↓	Ceramidase	–	+
Sphingosine			
↓	Sphingosine kinase	–	+
Sphingosine 1-phosphate			

Fig. 1.2. Sphingomyelin turnover and the enzymes responsible. Also shown are the enzymes that have been found to be activated (+) by cytokines such as TNFα and IL-1β or by growth factors, such as a platelet-derived growth factor.

Regulation of Gene Expression by Interleukin-1β (IL-1β) in Rat Hepatocytes

Inflammation results in numerous responses by the liver, which include the down-regulation by IL-1β of multiple P450 gene products, the synthesis of albumin and other so-called "negative acute-phase proteins," and the up-regulation of other genes such as that for α1-acid glycoprotein (AGP). We have recently shown that IL-1β induces the hydrolysis of sphingomyelin and accumulation of ceramide in hepatocytes; furthermore, the addition of short-chain ceramides or exogenous sphingomyelinase (to release endogenous ceramide) mimicked the effects of IL-1β on cytochrome P450-2C11 (CYP2C11) gene expression (5). These have become the standard criteria for assuming that the "sphingomyelin cycle" is involved in the response of cells to this cytokine (3). However, a number of our observations did not fit this model.

1. The time course of mass increase (5) (Fig. 1.3) in ceramide in response to IL-1β did not match the effects of this cytokine on suppression of CYP2C11 gene expression. In addition, the dose response for these two changes differed: Ceramide mass increased only with ≥5 ng/mL IL-1β, whereas 2.5–5 ng/mL IL-1β induced sphingomyelin turnover and suppression of CYP2C11 (5). On the other hand, the up-regulation of AGP and increase in ceramide mass exhibited the same IL-1β dosage dependence.

2. The dose response for down-regulation of CYP2C11 gene expression by short chain (C_2-) ceramide was lower than for the induction of AGP, which indicates that the regulation of these two genes does not proceed by the same pathway.

3. C_2-dihydroceramides were able to suppress CYP2C11 gene expression but were not able to induce AGP. The ceramide signaling pathway can usually be

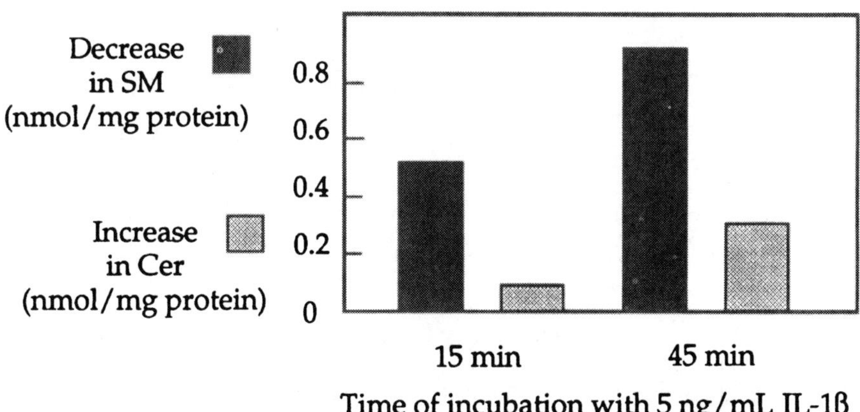

Fig. 1.3. Changes in the mass of sphingomyelin and ceramide after treatment of rat hepatocytes in culture with ≥5 ng/mL of IL-1β.

mimicked by C_2-ceramide but not by the saturated counterparts (i.e., C_2-dihydroceramides) (3).

We propose that the discrepancies between the regulation of CYP2C11 and AGP gene expression are explained by the utilization of more than one sphingolipid metabolite of sphingomyelin (as shown in Fig. 1.4): 2.5 ng/mL of IL-1β induces sphingomyelin hydrolysis to ceramide that is further cleaved to sphingosine and subsequent metabolites (which down-regulate CYP2C11), whereas at ≥5 ng/mL, IL-1β induces the hydrolysis of sphingomyelin to ceramide that undergoes little subsequent turnover (and induces the up-regulation of AGP). In recent studies (14), we have found that 2.5–5 ng/mL of IL-1β activates ceramidase whereas higher levels suppress ceramidase activity, which supports this hypothesis. As far as we are aware, this is the first time that such a bimodal regulation of this pathway has been suggested.

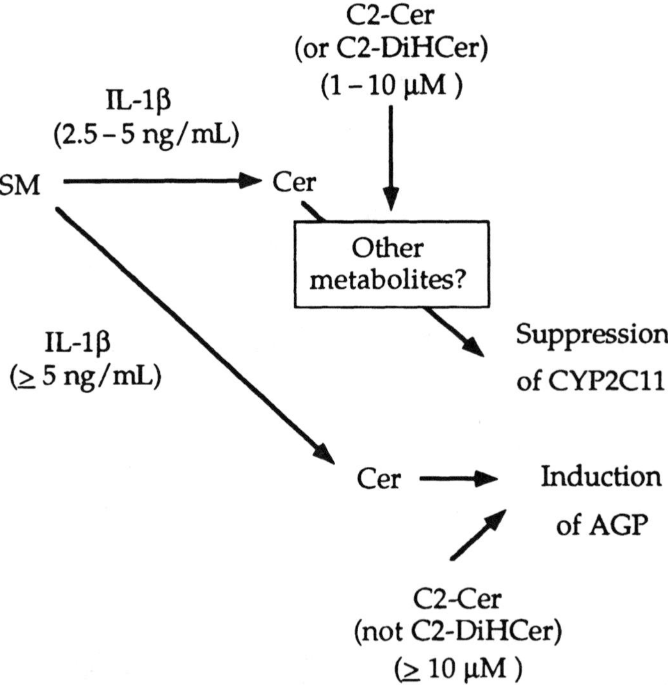

Fig. 1.4. A scheme summarizing the differences between down-regulation of cytochrome P450-2C11 (CYP2C11) and induction of α1–acid glycoprotein (AGP) by IL-1β in rat hepatocytes. The abbreviations are: Cer, ceramide; C2-Cer, N-acetylsphingosine; C2-DiHCer, N acetylsphinganine; SM, sphingomyelin.

Alteration of Sphingolipid Metabolism *In Vivo*

The potent and diverse biological activities of sphingosine, ceramide, and other sphingolipid metabolites in cell culture leads one to wonder about the *in vivo* consequences of altering sphingolipid metabolism or administration of the metabolites. This has been explored in only a few systems, but the findings are helping to explain the mechanisms of action of toxins and promise to provide new insight into the molecular basis for some of the relationships between diet and cancer.

Disruption of Sphingolipid Biosynthesis by Fumonisins

Fumonisins are a family of mycotoxins produced by *Fusarium moniliforme* (Sheldon) and related fungi that are common contaminants of corn (maize, *Zea mais*), sorghum, and related grains throughout the world (10). Animals that consume maize contaminated with *F. moniliforme* or purified fumonisins, such as the major species FB_1, can develop liver and kidney damage, severe neurotoxicity (equids), pulmonary edema (pigs), liver cancer, and other disease. These mycotoxins have also been implicated in human esophageal cancer in South Africa and China (16).

In 1991, FB_1 was shown to be a potent inhibitor of ceramide synthase and to block *de novo* sphingolipid biosynthesis (Fig. 1.5) (19). As a consequence of the inhibition of ceramide synthase, sphinganine accumulates in tissues, blood, and urine; furthermore, a substantial amount of sphinganine is diverted to sphinganine 1-phosphate and cleaved to fatty aldehydes and ethanolamine 1-phosphate. This route for ethanolamine phosphate synthesis has received little attention compared with the better known decarboxylation of phosphatidylserine, but it could make a significant contribution to the cellular ethanolamine pool (11).

The toxicity and carcinogenicity of fumonisins appear to involve both a loss of complex sphingolipid formation and an elevation in free sphingoid bases, the possible consequences of which have been summarized in Fig. 1.5 (11,15). In recent studies, we have found that sphingoid bases also undergo acetylation; therefore, it is possible that the formation of C_2 ceramide in animals exposed to FB_1 may contribute to the toxicity. Free sphingoid bases and ceramide individually, and in combination, can induce apoptosis (3), which FB_1 has also been shown to induce (11).

Inhibition of Colon Carcinogenesis by Dietary Sphingomyelin

Sphingolipids are hydrolyzed in the upper and lower gastrointestinal tract (16 and references cited therein) to ceramide and sphingosine (and possibly other metabolites), which are taken up by intestinal cells. Many types of cells in culture are now known to undergo changes in growth, differentiation, and apoptosis upon exposure to sphingoid bases or ceramides (12), and sphingosine and sphinganine have been shown to inhibit the transformation of C3H 10T1/2 cells exposed to γ irradiation and phorbol esters (4); therefore, we hypothesized that dietary sphingolipids might be able to inhibit colon carcinogenesis.

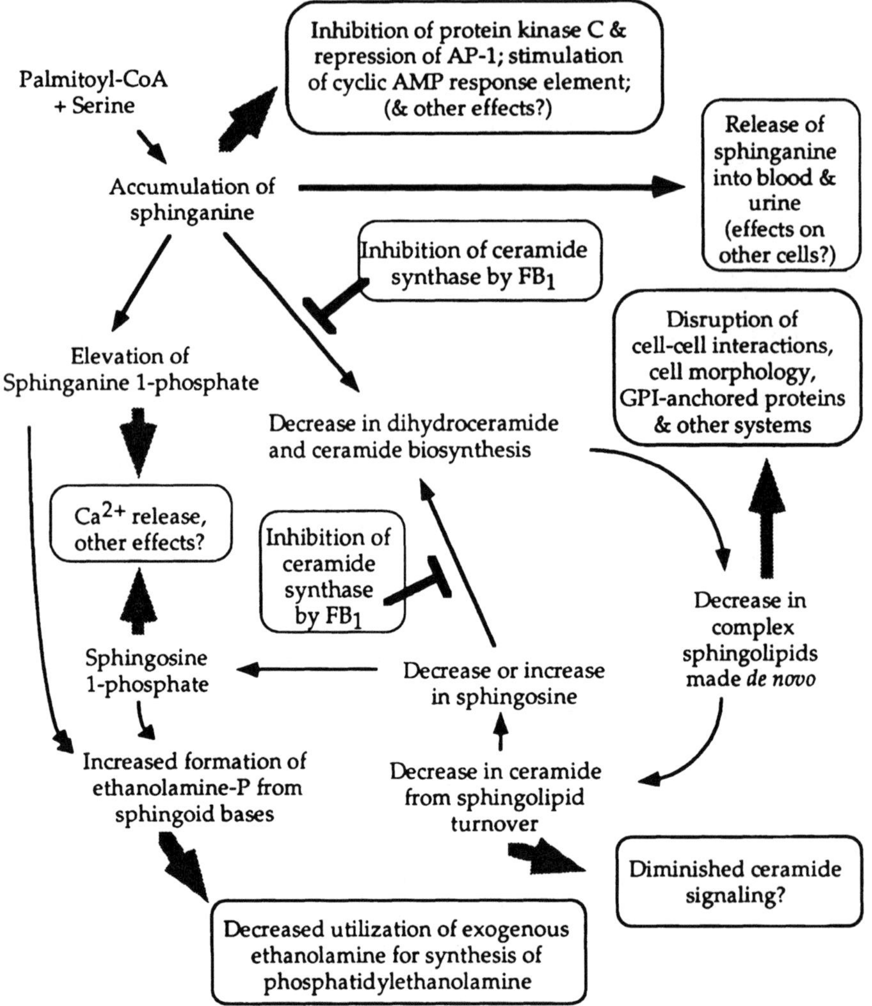

Fig. 1.5. A scheme summarizing the effects of fumonisin B_1 (FB_1) on sphingolipid metabolism, with the possible disruption of cell regulation as a consequence of these changes.

To test this hypothesis, female CF1 mice were treated with 1,2-dimethylhydrazine (DMH) (7) to induce colon tumors, then fed sphingomyelin (isolated from milk) in amounts ranging from 0.025 to 0.1% (w/w) of the diet, which is similar to the level in several foods (20). In a pilot study, sphingomyelin significantly reduced the number of aberrant colonic foci (an early marker of colon carcinogenesis) and decreased the number of animals with tumors, although the latter was only marginally significant due to the small number of animals tested (7).

In a follow-up investigation (17), sphingomyelin reduced the number of aberrant colonic crypt foci and the number of crypts per focus, and shifted the types of tumors induced by DMH from exclusively adenocarcinomas to a combination of adenomas and adenocarcinomas (Fig. 1.6). These findings suggest that sphingomyelin (presumably through its metabolism in the colon, with the possible involvement of colonic microflora) inhibits the promotion and/or progression of colon carcinogenesis; however, it is also possible that sphingolipids can induce differentiation or apoptosis in colon tumors.

A simple explanation for these effects may be that dietary sphingolipids deliver unusually high levels of these bioactive metabolites to colonic cells and thus have an essentially "pharmacologic" effect. However, the amounts of sphingomyelin that were fed are relatively small, and less than 10% escapes digestion and uptake by the upper intestine to appear in the colon. It is possible, therefore, that dietary sphingolipids are acting in amounts that are almost normal. This raises the possibility that

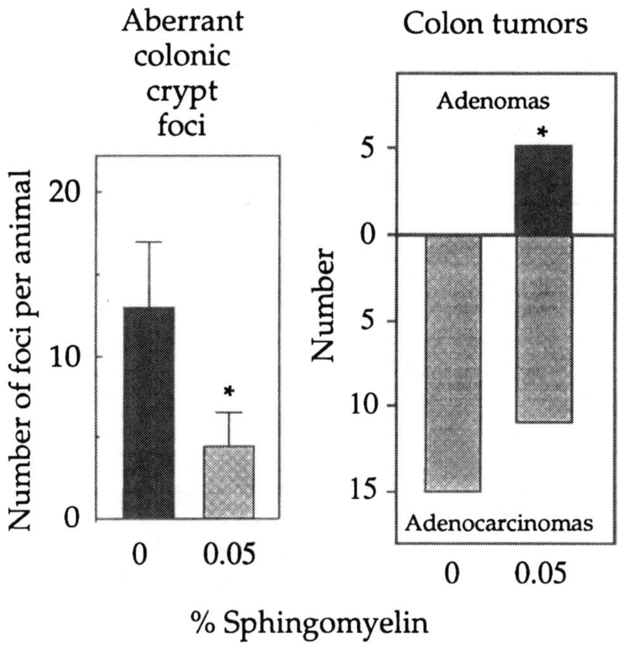

Fig. 1.6. Effects of sphingomyelin feeding on the number of aberrant colonic crypt foci (left panel) and the number of adenomas versus adenocarcinomas (right panel) in female CF1 mice administered 1,2-dimethylhydrazine. The asterisks indicate that the mice fed sphingomyelin were significantly ($P < 0.05$) different from the controls. Data are from Schmelz et al. (Ref. 17).

                    E.-M. Schmelz et al.

they are normalizing a defect in the ability of transformed cells to produce ceramide and/or sphingosine for cell signaling (Fig. 1.7). Although this seems speculative, others have noted that one of the first changes in rat colonic cells induced by DMH is a decrease in membrane fluidity that appears to be due to increases in membrane sphingomyelin. The elevation was associated with an increase in sphingomyelin synthesis and a reduction in the activity of the (neutral) sphingomyelinase [see discussion (17)]. Therefore, we propose that the suppression of colonic adenocarcinomas by dietary sphingolipids may reflect the restoration of a defective signaling event that is key to growth regulation, differentiation, and/or apoptosis. If this is the case, a better understanding of the consequences of delivering sphingolipids to tumors might be important, not only in understanding the relationships between diet and cancer but also for the development of new approaches to cancer chemotherapy.

Perspectives for the Future

Altogether these studies underscore the diverse and complex roles of sphingolipids as second messengers, as mediators of the action of toxins, and as potentially beneficial components of the diet. It is interesting to look at current textbooks of biochemistry and note that most mention only the relationships between sphin-

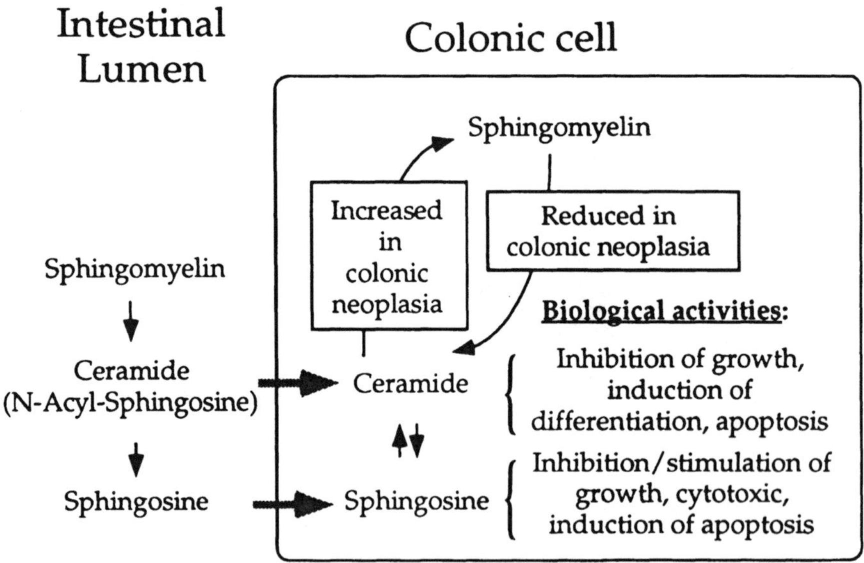

Fig. 1.7. A model for the effects of dietary sphingomyelin on colon carcinogenesis, also illustrating the possibility of defect(s) in sphingomyelin metabolism that might affect the amounts of endogenous ceramide and other bioactive metabolites.

golipids and disease are the sphingolipidoses caused by genetic defects in sphingolipid hydrolases, whereas work over the past decade has established that

- Sphingolipids are mediators of the effects of cholera toxin, verotoxin, and viruses that bind to intestinal cells *via* glycolipids.

- Disruption of sphingolipid metabolism by fumonisins causes a wide variety of diseases of agricultural animals and perhaps humans.

- There are, in fact, many naturally occurring inhibitors of sphingolipid metabolism, such as *Alternaria* toxins, australifungins, lipoxamycin, sphingofungins, and ISP-1 or myriocin (reviewed in ref. 12), that could play a role in disease.

- There is a considerable likelihood that some diseases (including cancer) involve aberrant sphingolipid signaling.

These new aspects of sphingolipidology offer tremendous potential for biomedical research, from the development of new pharmaceuticals to the design of functional foods for the prevention of disease.

References

1. Barenholz, Y. and Thompson, T.E. (1980) Sphingomyelins in Bilayers and Biological Membranes, *Biochim. Biophys. Acta 604*, 129–158.
2. Bell, R.M., Hannun, Y.A., and Merrill, A.H., Jr. (1993) *Advances in Lipid Research: Sphingolipids and Their Metabolites,* Vol. 25–26, Academic Press, Orlando, FL.
3. Bielawska, A., Linardic, C.M., and Hannun, Y.A. (1992) Ceramide-Mediated Biology: Determination of Structural and Stereospecific Requirements through the Use of N-Acyl -Phenylaminoalcohol Analogs, *J. Biol. Chem. 267*, 18493–18497.
4. Borek, C., Ong, A., Stevens, V.L., Wang, E., and Merrill, A.H., Jr. (1991) Long-Chain (Sphingoid) Bases Inhibit Multistage Carcinogenesis in Mouse C3H/10T1/2 Cells Treated with Radiation and Phorbol 12-Myristate 13-Acetate, *Proc. Natl. Acad. Sci. USA 88*, 1953–1957.
5. Chen, J., Nikolova-Karakashian, M., Merrill, A.H., Jr., and Morgan, E.T. (1995) Regulation of Cytochrome P450 2CII (CYP2C11) Gene Expression by Interleukin-1, Sphingomyelin Hydrolysis, and Ceramides in Rat Hepatocytes, *J. Biol. Chem. 270*, 25233–25238.
6. Coroneos, E., Martinez, M., McKenna, S., and Kester, M. (1995) Differential Regulation of Sphingomyelinase and Ceramidase Activities by Growth Factors and Cytokines— Implications for Cellular Proliferation and Differentiation, *J. Biol. Chem. 270*, 23305–23309.
7. Dillehay, D.L., Webb, S.J., Schmelz, E.-M., and Merrill, A.H., Jr. (1994) Dietary Sphingomyelin Inhibits 1,2-Dimethylhydrazine-Induced Colon Cancer in CF1 Mice, *J. Nutr. 124*, 615–620.
8. Hannun, Y.A. (1994) The Sphingomyelin Cycle and the Second Messenger Function of Ceramide, *J. Biol. Chem. 269*, 3125–3128.
9. Kolesnick, R., and Golde, D.W. (1994) The Sphingomyelin Pathway in Tumor Necrosis Factor and Interleukin-1 Signaling, *Cell 77*, 325–328.
10. Marasas, W.F.O. (1982) Mycotoxicological Investigations on Corn Produced in

Oesophageal Cancer Areas in Transkei, in *Cancer of the Oesophagus*, C.J. Pfeiffer, ed., CRC Press, Boca Raton, Florida, vol. 1, pp. 29–40.

11. Merrill, A.H., Jr., Liotta, D.C., and Riley, R.E. (1996) Fumonisins: Fungal Toxins That Shed Light on Sphingolipid Function. *Trends Cell Biol. 6*, 218–223.

12. Merrill, A.H., Jr., Liotta, D.C., and Riley, R.E., Bioactive Properties of Sphingosine and Structurally Related Compounds, in *Handbook of Lipid Research,* Bell, R.M., Exton, J.H., and Prescott, S.M., eds., Plenum Press, New York, 8, 205–237.

13. Merrill, A.H., Jr., and Sweeley, C.C. (1996) Sphingolipids: Metabolism and Cell Signalling, in *New Comprehensive Biochemistry: Biochemistry of Lipids, Lipoproteins, and Membranes,* Vance, D.E., and Vance, J.E., eds., Elsevier, Amsterdam, vol. 31, pp. 309–338.

14. Nikolova-Karakashian, M., Morgan, E.T., Alexander, C., Liotta, D.C., and Merrill, A.H., Jr. (1997) Bimodal Regulation of Ceramidase by Interleukin-1β, *J. Biol. Chem. 272*, 18718–18724.

15. Riley, R.T., Voss, K.A., Yoo, H.-S., Gelderblom, W.C.A., and Merrill, A.H. Jr. (1994) Mechanism of Fumonisin Toxicity and Carcinogenicity, *J. Food Protect. 57*, 638–645.

16. Schmelz, E.-M., Crall, K.J., LaRocque, R., Dillehay, D.L., and Merrill, A.H., Jr. (1994) Uptake and Metabolism of Sphingolipids in Isolated Intestinal Loops of Mice, *J. Nutr. 124*, 702–712.

17. Schmelz, E.-M., Dillehay, D.L., Webb, S.K., Reiter, A., Adams, J., and Merrill, A.H., Jr. (1996) Sphingomyelin Consumption Suppresses Aberrant Colonic Crypt Foci and Increases the Proportion of Adenomas versus Adenocarcinomas in CF1 Mice Treated with 1,2-Dimethylhydrazine. *Cancer Res. 56*, 4936–4941.

18. Spiegel, S., and Merrill, A.H., Jr. (1996) Sphingolipid Metabolism and Growth Regulation: A State-of-the-Art Review. *FASEB J. 10*, 1388–1397.

19. Wang, E., Norred, W.P., Bacon, C.W., Riley, R.T., and Merrill, A.H., Jr. (1991) Inhibition of Sphingolipid Biosynthesis by Fumonisins. Implications for Diseases Associated with *Fusarium moniliforme. J. Biol. Chem. 266*, 14486–14490.

20. Zeisel, S.H., Char, D., and Sheard, N.F. (1986) Choline, Phosphatidylcholine and Sphingomyelin in Human and Bovine Milk and Infant Formulas, *J. Nutr. 116*, 50–58.

Chapter 2

Choline Phospholipids and Cell Suicide

Chi-Liang E. Yen and Steven H. Zeisel

Department of Nutrition, School of Public Health, School of Medicine, CB#7400, University of North Carolina, Chapel Hill, NC 27599-7400

Introduction

Choline phospholipids play major roles in cellular regulation in addition to their essential function as structural components of membranes and lipoproteins. We review the involvement of choline phospholipids in signal transduction pathways, especially those related to cell death.

Functions of Choline and Choline Phospholipids

Choline is a dietary component that is the major source of methyl groups in the diet and is the precursor of the neurotransmitter acetylcholine (1). Most choline in the body is found in phospholipids. The choline phospholipids ensure the structural integrity and signaling functions of cell membranes and are vital for lipid transport (1). Phosphatidylcholine is the predominant phospholipid (>50%) in most mammalian membranes. Though representing a smaller proportion of the total choline pool, other choline phospholipids are important, including sphingomyelin, platelet-activating factor, choline plasmalogens, and lysophosphatidylcholine.

Phospholipids and Signal Transduction

It is crucial for cells to be able to communicate with and respond to their environment. Phospholipids and their metabolites have an important role in these signaling processes (2). In a simplified view, stimulation of membrane-associated receptors activates neighboring phospholipases, resulting in the formation of breakdown products of phospholipids that are signaling molecules either by themselves (i.e., they stimulate or inhibit the activity of target macromolecules), or after conversion to signaling molecules by specific enzymes.

Phospholipid signaling research once focused on phosphatidylinositol derivatives; this research is extensively reviewed elsewhere (3,4). We now realize that choline phospholipids, especially phosphatidylcholine and sphingomyelin, are also substrates for formation of biologically active molecules that can amplify external signals or that can terminate the signaling process by generating inhibitory second messengers (5–7).

In some phospholipid signaling processes, activation of receptors at the plasma membrane leads to altered conformation of the receptor so that it can activate a GTP-binding protein (G protein). The activation of the G protein results in the subsequent activation of phospholipase C activity within the plasma membrane. The phospholipase Cs are a family of phosphodiesterases that hydrolyze the glycerophosphate bond of intact phospholipids to generate 1,2-*sn*-diacylglycerol and an aqueous soluble head group. Numerous phosphatidylinositol bisphosphate-specific phospholipase Cs exist, and specific receptors couple to specific phospholipase C isotypes (8). In a similar manner, specific receptors appear to be linked to activation of specific phosphatidylcholine phospholipase Cs, generating diacylglycerol (DAG), which sustains cascades of messengers first initiated by the breakdown of phosphatidylinositol bisphosphate (5).

The action of phospholipase C catalyzes the next event in the signal cascade, which is the activation of protein kinase C (PKC; serine/threonine kinase). Products generated by phosphatidylcholine hydrolysis include diacylglycerol, which is both a messenger molecule and an intermediate in the metabolism of lipids (9). Normally, conventional PKC is folded so that an endogenous "pseudosubstrate" region on the protein is bound to the catalytic site, thereby inhibiting activity. Diacylglycerol causes a conformational change in PKC, causing flexing at a hinge region so as to withdraw the pseudosubstrate and unblock the PKC catalytic site (2,5). Multiple PKC isoforms have been identified so far. They are categorized into three groups (10): conventional PKCs (α, $\beta1$, $\beta2$, and γ), novel PKCs (δ, ε, η, θ, and μ), and atypical PKCs (ζ, λ, and ι). This categorization is based on whether a specific isoform can be activated by Ca^{2+} and diacylglycerol. Novel PKCs bind to phorbol esters and thus can be activated by diacylglycerol, while the activation is independent of Ca^{2+} (they lack the second constant region of the PKC protein, C2). Atypical PKCs lack the C2 region and possess only one of the two zinc finger regions found in the other PKCs; they do not bind to phorbol ester or diacylglycerol, and their activation is Ca^{2+}-independent. It is possible that different combinations of lipid second messengers transduce signals for unique cell functions by activating specific subsets of PKC isoforms.

The characterization of events that occur downstream from PKC is just beginning. Serine-threonine kinases and tyrosine kinases catalyze phosphorylation of target proteins distal to PKC. Phosphorylation alters the biochemical properties of these substrates, resulting in a range of cellular responses. These phosphorylation cascades serve to enhance amplification of the original signal. The targets for phosphorylation by PKC include receptors for insulin, epidermal growth factor, and many proteins involved in control of gene expression (4,11,12).

Other products of phosphatidylcholine hydrolysis, such as phosphatidic acid, lysophosphatidylcholine, and free fatty acids also are second messengers (5). Phosphatidic acid can act as a mitogen (13). Lysophosphatidylcholine stimulates PKC activity (14) and is important in chemotaxis, relaxation of smooth muscle, and activation of T-lymphocytes. Arachidonic acid is a precursor of prostaglandins (15).

Although sphingolipids are ubiquitous components of mammalian cells, it has only recently been proven that their metabolism generates intracellular second messengers (ceramide, sphingosine, sphingosine 1-phosphate, and sphingosylphosphocholine) that regulate cell growth, differentiation, and programmed cell death (7,16–19). A number of extracellular agents, such as vitamin D_3, tumor necrosis factor (TNF)-α, and corticosteroids, evoke sphingomyelinase activity (7,20–22). Activation of sphingomyelinase (sphingomyelin-specific phospholipase C) increases cleavage of sphingomyelin, generating ceramide, a compound with potent biological activities including the induction of programmed cell death (apoptosis) (23). Ceramide is a substrate for sphingomyelin synthase (phosphatidylcholine-ceramide phosphocholine transferase) as shown in Fig. 2.1, reaction 1 (24). Ceramide can also be phosphorylated to form ceramide 1-phosphate (Fig. 2.1, reaction 4) (25) by a calcium-dependent kinase (26).

Other sphingomyelin-derived molecules include those that induce mitosis (sphingosine-P, sphingosylphosphocholine) (27,28) or growth arrest (sphingosine) (7) (Fig. 2.1, reactions 6 and 7).

Sphingosine, intermediate of both biosynthesis and turnover of ceramide, is growth-inhibitory and cytotoxic (29). Sphingosine is a potent inhibitor of PKC that acts by blocking diacylglycerol-mediated activation (24). Further, sphingosine's inhibition of phosphatidic acid phosphohydrolase (an enzyme that generates the PKC-activator diacylglycerol) diminishes activation of PKC (30,31). Direct activation of diacylglycerol kinase by sphingosine also removes diacylglycerol (32). Sphingosine is also an apoptosis inducer in HL-60 cells (33), and it potentiates ceramide-mediated cytotoxicity (34). Sphingosine stimulates growth of some types of cells in a PKC-independent manner (35,36).

Sphingosylphosphocholine, also formed during hydrolysis of sphingomyelin, inhibits PKC (37). In addition, sphingosylphosphocholine is a potent mitogen (27,28).

Sphingosine 1-phosphate, a metabolite of ceramide, is mitogenic (38) and has been implicated as second messenger in cell proliferation induced by platelet-derived growth factor and serum (39,40). It prevents apoptosis caused by ceramide (41). It has been proposed that the dynamic balance between levels of sphingosine

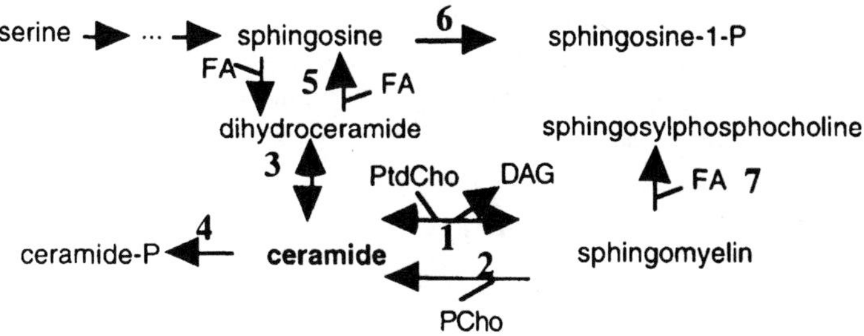

Fig.2.1. Pathways for ceramide generation.

1-phosphate and ceramide may be important for determining whether a cell survives or undergoes apoptosis (41,42).

There are several instances in which phosphatidylcholine and sphingomyelin hydrolysis are activated sequentially in a signaling pathway. For example, tumor necrosis factor (TNF) induces the activation of a phosphatidylcholine-specific phospholipase C and the activation of cytosolic phospholipase A_2 (43). The lipid messengers, diacylglycerol and arachidonic acid, produced by these phospholipases are selective activators of a lysosomal/endosomal acidic sphingomyelinase and a neutral cytosolic sphingomyelinase, respectively. As another example, the Fas/APO-1 death factor receptor induces sequential activation of phosphatidylcholine-specific phospholipase C and acidic sphingomyelinase (44); perhaps this is a regulatory counterbalancing mechanism. Activation of protein kinase C counterbalances apoptotic signals induced by TNF-α, Fas ligand, and ionizing radiation, suggesting that the DAG/PKC pathway counteracts ceramide-mediated apoptosis (23,45,46). Conversely, PKC-ζ is bifunctionally regulated by ceramide and arachidonic acid (47).

More about Programmed Cell Death (Apoptosis)

Programmed cell death, also called apoptosis, is an essential regulatory mechanism by which unwanted and damaged cells can be eliminated during normal development and tissue homeostasis. Apoptosis is a regulated form of cell suicide (48) in which cells activate endonuclease activity that cleaves transcriptionally active nuclear DNA into internucleosomal fragments of 200-base-pair length (forming a "ladder" on gel electrophoresis) (49,50). These cells are recognized by characteristic morphological features (51,52). We now recognize that highly regulated, internally encoded suicide programs also play a major role in many diseases, including cancer (53,54), acquired immunodeficiency syndrome (55), heart disease (56), and neurodegenerative disorders (57,58). A wide variety of signals induces or inhibits apoptosis (59). These signals may converge on a central common cell execution process. Genes found to regulate this final common cell death pathway are conserved across evolution, from worms to humans (48,60,61). For example, inter-leukin-1β-converting enzyme (ICE)–related cysteine proteases, which are the mammalian homologs of the *Caenorhabditis elegans* cell death protein ced-3, are required for the execution of apoptosis induced by several different stimuli (62,63). Knowledge on how apoptosis can be modulated could lead to development of treatments and/or prevention applications for a variety of significant diseases.

Choline Deficiency and Cell Death

Though it has been proposed that choline deficiency kills liver cells because they accumulate massive amounts of fat and rupture their plasma membranes (64), we have observed that choline-deficient hepatocytes begin to die long before lipid accumulation threatens membrane integrity (54,65,66). Choline deficiency, in both rats and cultured cells, induces apoptosis. For example, rat hepatocytes in which p53 tumor suppressor protein is inactivated respond by inducing free radical-dependent apoptosis when acutely switched to a medium containing low choline (65). Choline deficiency is a potent apoptosis inducer in neuronal cells as well. Using PC12 cells (a neuronal cell line derived from a rat pheochromocytoma), we were able to show that choline deficiency could turn on apoptotic death, with characteristic DNA strand breaks and apoptotic body formation (67).

Choline deficiency-induced apoptosis occurs via a pathway that involves reactive oxygen species as intermediates (54,65). Neocuproine prevents hydroxyl radical formation and was more effective in suppressing choline deficiency-induced apoptosis than was N-acetylcysteine, which traps free radicals after they are formed (68). Reactive oxygen species (ROS) are involved in several described apoptosis signaling pathways (69). H_2O_2-induced apoptosis is a popular model system (70,71). A suggested mechanism of action for Bcl-2, an apoptosis suppressor protein, is that it regulates an antioxidant pathway at sites of free radical generation (72). Production of ROS has been previously described in rats fed a choline-deficient (CD) diet, and these ROS caused DNA damage (8-hydroxyguanosine residues) (73).

We have previously reported that choline deficiency-induced apoptosis occurs because of a deficiency in choline moieties rather than because of methyl deficiency (66). Death was directly correlated with cellular phosphatidylcholine concentration (54), and several other investigators suggest that phosphatidylcholine is a critical molecule that is associated with apoptosis (74–76). Perhaps this is because phosphatidylcholine synthesis is also needed for progression of the cell cycle (77,78).

Ceramide concentrations increase in PC12 cells deprived of choline at about the same time that cellular phosphatidylcholine concentrations decrease (unpublished data)—crossing a threshold level that we have previously demonstrated to be highly correlated with induction of apoptosis in hepatocytes (54). Ceramide, derived from the choline phospholipid sphingomyelin as discussed above, plays a key antiproliferative role in cells exposed to environmental stress, including those signal inducers leading to apoptosis, cell cycle arrest, and cell senescence (7). Most of the inducers of apoptosis, terminal differentiation, or growth suppression also induce ceramide accumulation (79), which precedes the cellular effects of these extracellular agents. In addition, cell-permeable analogs of ceramide, such as C_2- and C_6-ceramide, mimic the effects of extracellular inducers that raise ceramide levels (23). Exogenously added C_2-ceramide could induce apoptosis in PC12 cells (80). Ceramide mediates apoptosis through a stress-activated protein kinase (SAPK/JNK) and caspases (ICE-related proteinase) (79,81). Other candidates for mediators of ceramide action include ceramide-activated phosphatase, PKC-ζ, and ceramide-activated protein kinase (7).

1-*O*-alkyl-2-acetyl-*sn*-glycero-3-phosphocholine (platelet-activating factor, PAF) is another choline phospholipid that is involved in apoptosis signaling in some types of cells. It abrogated apoptosis in a human B lymphoblastoid cell line (82); it induced apoptosis in cultured hippocampal neurons (N. Bazan, abstract presented at Eicosanoids Conference 9/97); and it induced apoptosis when it was added to CEM-C12 human *T* cells in the presence of calcium ionophore (83). We do not know how choline deficiency affects PAF levels.

We found that hepatocytes can be adapted so that they can survive in a low-choline medium by becoming resistant to choline deficiency-induced apoptosis (54). Adapted cells did not survive because they corrected intracellular concentrations of choline or water-soluble choline metabolites; however, adapted cells did slightly increase intracellular phosphatidylcholine concentrations compared to acutely deficient cells (54). This increase in phosphatidylcholine concentration could be the result of enhanced endogenous production of phosphatidylcholine *via* the methylation of phosphatidylethanolamine. This observation is consistent with the reports that the activity of PtdEtn-*N*-methyltransferase activity is increased in the livers of choline-deficient rats (84).

Choline Deficiency in Humans

Humans can become depleted of choline and develop liver damage when fed purified diets (84) or when fed parenterally with low-choline formulations (86–88). In choline-deficient rats there is enhanced hepatocyte cell death (89), compensatory increases in hepatocyte DNA synthesis, and liver regeneration (90). After 6 months on a choline-deficient diet, foci of preneoplastic hepatocytes appear in rat liver, and hepatocellular carcinomas occur at approximately 12 months, despite the absence of any known carcinogens (91). The mechanism for the cancer-promoting effect of choline deficiency is not completely elucidated. Perturbations in important intracellular signaling mechanisms regulating cell growth involving hepatic 1,2-*sn*-diacylglycerol concentration and protein kinase C (PKC) activity occur in choline deficiency (92). The chronic cell death and cell proliferation in choline-deficient liver, with its associated increased rate of DNA synthesis, could cause greater sensitivity to chemical carcinogens (93). Alterations in the genome that occur in choline deficiency, such as hypomethylation of DNA (90,94–96) and DNA damage caused by free radicals (97,98), also probably enhance carcinogenesis. We add to this list of mechanisms the possibility that loss of an apoptosis pathway contributes to carcinogenesis in the liver of choline-deficient rats.

Summary

Choline phospholipids play major roles in cellular regulation in addition to their essential function as structural components of membranes and lipoproteins. The unique functions of choline phospholipids as hormones (platelet-activating factor) and sources of second messengers (phosphatidylcholine, sphingomyelin) may explain how dietary choline influences normal physiological processes as well as a diverse group of pathological processes including carcinogenesis.

Acknowledgments

This work was funded by a grant from the NIH (AG09525) to Dr. Zeisel. Mr. Yen is the recipient of a graduate fellowship from the Chinook Company.

References

1. Zeisel, S.H., and Blusztajn, J.K. (1994) Choline and Human Nutrition, *Annu. Rev. Nutr. 14*, 269–296.
2. Zeisel, S.H. (1993) Choline Phospholipids: Signal Transduction and Carcinogenesis, *FASEB J. 7*, 551–557.
3. Exton, J.H., Taylor, S.J., Blank, J.S., and Bocckino, S.B. (1992) Regulation of Phosphoinositide and Phosphatidylcholine Phospholipases by G Proteins, *Ciba Found. Symp. 164*, 36–42.
4. Nishizuka, Y. (1995) Protein Kinase C and Lipid Signaling for Sustained Cellular Responses, *FASEB J. 9*, 484–496.
5. Exton, J.H. (1994) Phosphatidylcholine Breakdown and Signal Transduction, *Biochim. Biophys. Acta 1212*, 26–42.
6. Zeisel, S. (1995) Nutrients, Signal Transduction and Carcinogenesis, *Adv. Exper. Med. Biol. 369*, 175–83.
7. Hannun, Y. (1996) Functions of Ceramide in Coordinating Cellular Responses to Stress, *Science 274*, 1855–1859.
8. Meldrum, E., Parker, P.J., and Carozzi, A. (1991) The Ptd-Ins-PLC Superfamily and Signal Transduction, *Biochim. Biophys. Acta 1092*, 49–71.
9. Besterman, J.M., Duronio, V., and Cuatrecasas, P. (1986) Rapid Formation of Diacylglycerol from Phosphatidylcholine: A Pathway for Generation of a Second Messenger, *Proc. Natl. Acad. Sci. USA 83*, 6785–6789.
10. Newton, A.C. (1997) Regulation of Protein Kinase C, *Curr. Opin. Cell Biol. 9*, 161–167.
11. Jaken, S. (1996) Protein Kinase C Isozymes and Substrates, *Curr. Opin. Cell Biol. 8*, 168–173.
12. Gallicano, G., Yousef, M., and Capco, D. (1997) PKC—A Pivotal Regulator of Early Development, *Bioessays 19*, 29–36.
13. Wakelam, M.J.O., Cook, S.J., Currie, S., Plamer, S., and Plevin, R. (1991) Regulation of the Hydrolysis of Phosphatidylcholine in Swiss 3T3 Cells, *Biochem. Soc. Trans. 19*, 321–324.
14. Nishizuka, Y. (1992) Intracellular Signaling by Hydrolysis of Phospholipids and Activation of Protein Kinase C, *Science 258*, 607–614.
15. Lands, W.E.M. (1992) Biochemistry and Physiology of n-3 Fatty Acids, *FASEB J. 6*, 2530–2536.
16. Merrill, A.H. (1992) Ceramide: A New Lipid "Second Messenger"? *Nutr. Rev. 50*, 78–80.
17. Hannun, Y.A. (1994) The Sphingomyelin Cycle and the Second Messenger Function of Ceramide, *J. Biol. Chem. 269*, 3125–3128.
18. Spiegel, S., and Merrill, A.J. (1996) Sphingolipid Metabolism and Cell Growth Regulation, *FASEB J. 10*, 1388–1397.
19. Sun, L., Xu, L., Henry, F., Spiegel, S., and Nielsen, T. (1996) A New Wound Healing Agent—Sphingosylphosphorycholine, *J. Invest. Dermatol. 106*, 232–237.

20. Okazaki, T., Bielawska, A., Bell, R.M.. and Hannun, Y.A. (1990) Role of Ceramide as a Lipid Mediator of la,25-Dihydroxyvitamin D3–Induced HL-60 Cell Differentiation, *J. Biol. Chem. 265,* 15823–15831.

21. Ramachandran, C.K., Murray, D.K., and Nelson, D.H. (1990) Dexamethasone Increases Neutral Sphingomyelinase Activity and Sphingosine Levels in 3T3-L1 Fibroblasts, *Biochem. Biophys. Res. Commun. 167,* 607–613.

22. Dressler, K.A., Mathias, S., and Kolesnick, R.N. (1992) Tumor Necrosis Factor-α Activates the Sphingomyelin Signal Transduction Pathway in a Cell-Free System, *Science 255,* 1715–1718.

23. Obeid, L.M., Linardic, C.M., Karolak, L.A.. and Hannun, Y.A. (1993) Programmed Cell Death Induced by Ceramide, *Science 259,* 1769–1771.

24. Merrill, A.H., and Jones, D.D. (1990) An Update of the Enzymology and Regulation of Sphingomyelin Metabolism, *Biochim. Biophys. Acta 1044,* 1–12.

25. Dressler, K.A., and Kolesnick, R.N. (1990) Ceramide 1-Phosphate, a Novel Phospholipid in Human Leukemia (HL-60) Cells. Synthesis via Ceramide from Sphingomyelin, *J. Biol. Chem. 265,* 14917–14921.

26. Kolesnick, R.N., and Hemer, M.R. (1990) Characterization of a Ceramide Kinase Activity from Human Leukemia (HL-60) Cells. Separation from Diacylglycerol Kinase Activity, *J. Biol. Chem. 265,* 18803–18808.

27. Desai, N.N., and Spiegel, S. (1991) Sphingosylphosphorylcholine Is a Remarkably Potent Mitogen for a Variety of Cell Lines, *Biochem. Biophys. Res. Commun. 181,* 361–366.

28. Desai, N.N., Carlson, R.0., Mattie, M.E., Olivera, A., Buckley, N.E., Seh, T., Brooker, G., and Spiegel, S. (1993) Signaling Pathways for Sphingosylphosphorylcholine-Mediated Mitogenesis in Swiss 3T3 Fibroblasts, *J. Cell. Biol. 121,* 1385–1395.

29. Merrill, A.H., Jr., Liotta, D.C., and Riley, R.E. (1995) Bioactive Properties of Sphingosine and Structurally Related Compounds, *Handb. Lipid Res. 8,* 205–237.

30. Liscovitch, M. (1991) Single-Dependent Activation of Phosphatidylcholine Hydrolysis: Role of Phospholipase D, *Biochem. Soc. Trans. 19,* 402–407.

31. Gomez-Munoz, A., Hamza, E.H., and Brindley, D.N. (1992) Effects of Sphingosine, Albumin and Unsaturated Fatty Acids on the Activation and Translocation of Phosphatidate Phosphohydrolases in Rat Hepatocytes, *Biochim. Biophys. Acta 1127,* 49–56.

32. Sakane, F., Yamada, K., and Kanoh, H. (1989) Different Effects of Sphingosine, R59022 and Anionic Amphiphiles on Two Diacylglycerol Kinase Isozymes Purified from Porcine Thymus Cytosol, *FEBS Lett. 255,* 409–413.

33. Skakura, C., Sweeney, E.A., Shirahama, T., Hakomori, S., and Igarashi, Y. (1996) Suppression of bcl-2 Gene Expression by Sphingosine in the Apoptosis of Human Leukemic HL-60 Cells During Phorbol Ester-Induced Terminal Differentiation, *FEBS Lett. 379,* 177–180.

34. Jarvis, W.D., Fornari, F.A., Jr., Traylor, R.S., Martin, H.A., Kramer, L.B., and Grant, G. (1996) Induction of Apoptosis and Potentiation of Ceramide-Mediated Cytotoxicity by Sphingoid Bases in Human Myeloid Leukemia Cells, *J. Biol. Chem. 271,* 8275–8284.

35. Zhang, H., Buckley, N.E., Gibson, K., and Spiegel, S. (1990) Sphingosine Stimulates Cellular Proliferation via a Protein Kinase C-Independent Pathway, *J. Biol. Chem. 265,* 76–81.

36. Jacobs, L.S., and Kester, M. (1993) Sphingolipids as Mediators of Effects of Platelet-Derived Growth Factor in Vascular Smooth Muscle, *Am. J. Physiol. 65,* c740–c747.

37. Hannun, Y.A., and Bell, R.M. (1989) Regulation of Protein Kinase C by Sphingosine and Lysosphingolipids, *Clin. Chim. Acta 185,* 333–345.
38. Spiegel, S., and Milstien, S. (1995) Sphingolipid Metabolites: Members of a New Class of Lipid Second Messengers, *J. Memb. Biol. 146,* 225–37.
39. Olivera, A., and Spiegel, S. (1993) Sphingosine-1-Phosphate as Second Messenger in Cell Proliferation Induced by PDGF and FCS Mitogens, *Nature 365,* 557–560.
40. Coroneos, E., Martinez, M., Mckenna, S., and Kester, M. (1995) Differential Regulation of Sphingomyelinase and Ceramidase Activities by Growth Factors and Cytokines, *J. Biol. Chem. 270,* 23305–23309.
41. Cuvillier, O., Pirianov, G., Kleuser, B., Vanek, P.G., Coso, O.A., and Spiegel, S. (1996) Suppression of Ceramide-Mediated Programmed Cell Death by Sphingosine-1-phosphate, *Nature 381,* 800–803.
42. Xia, Z., Dickens, M., Raingeaud, J., Davis, R., and Greenberg, M. (1995) Opposing Effects of ERK and JNK-p38 MAP Kinases on Apoptosis, *Science 270,* 1326–1331.
43. Heller, R., and Kronke, M. (1994) Tumor Necrosis Factor Receptor-Mediated Signaling Pathways, *J. Cell Biol. 126,* 5–9.
44. Cifone, M., Roncaioli, P., De Maria, R., Camarda, G., Santoni, A., Ruberti, G., and Testi, R. (1995) Multiple Pathways Originate at the Fas/APO-1 (CD95) Receptor: Sequential Involvement of Phosphatidylcholine-Specific Phospholipase C and Acidic Sphingomyelinase in the Propagation of the Apoptotic Signal, *EMBO J. 14,* 5859–5868.
45. Jarvis, W., Fornari, F., Browning, J., Gewirtz, D., Kolesnick, R., and Grant, S. (1994) Attenu- ation of Ceramide-Induced Apoptosis by Diglyceride in Human Myeloid Leukemia Cells, *J. Biol. Chem. 269,* 31685–31692.
46. Tepper, C., Jayadev, S., Liu, B., Bielawska, A., Wolff, R., Yonehara, S., Hannun, Y., and Seldin, M. (1995) Role for Ceramide as an Endogenous Mediator of Fas-Induced Cytotoxicity, *Proc. Natl. Acad. Sci. USA 92,* 8443–8447.
47. Muller, G., Ayoub, M., Storz, P., Rennecke, J., Fabbro, D., and Pfizenmaier, K. (1995) PKC zeta Is a Molecular Switch in Signal Transduction of TNF-alpha Bifunctionally Regulated by Ceramide and Arachidonic Acid, *EMBO J. 14,* 1961–1969.
48. Schwartzman, R.A., and Cidlowski, J.A. (1993) Apoptosis: The Biochemistry and Molecular Biology of Programmed Cell Death, *Endoc. Rev. 14,* 133–151.
49. Kokileva, L. (1994) Multi-Step Chromatin Degradation in Apoptosis, *Int. Arch. Allergy Immunol. 105,* 339–343.
50. Zhivotovsky, B., Wade, D., Nicotera, P., and Orrenius, S. (1994) Role of Nucleases in Apoptosis, *Int. Arch. Allergy Immunol. 105,* 333–338.
51. Wyllie, A.H. (1987) Cell Death, *Int. Rev. Cytol. 17* (Suppl), 755–785.
52. Arends, M.J., Morris, R.G., and Wyllie, A.H. (1990) Apoptosis. The Role of the Endonuclease, *Am. J. Pathol. 136,* 593–608.
53. Martikainen, P., Kyprianou, N., Tucker, R.W., and Isaacs, J.T. (1991) Programmed Death of Nonproliferating Androgen-Independent Prostatic Cancer Cells, *Cancer Res. 51,* 4693–4700.
54. Zeisel, S.H., Albright, C.D., Shin, O.-K., Mar, M.-H., Salganik, R.I., and da Costa, K.-A. (1997) Choline Deficiency Selects for Resistance to p53-Independent Apoptosis and Causes Tumorigenic Transformation of Rat Hepatocytes, *Carcinogenesis 18,* 731–738.
55. Adle-Biassette, H., Levy, Y., Colombel, M., Poron, F., Natchev, S., Keohane, C., and Gray, F. (1995) Neuronal Apoptosis in HIV Infection in Adults, *Neuropathol. Appl. Neurobiol. 21,* 218–227.

56. Olivetti, G., Abbi, R., Quaini, F., Kajstura, J., Cheng, W., Nitahara, J., Quaini, E., Di Loreto, C., Beltrami, C., Krajewski, S., Reed, J., and Anversa, P. (1997) Apoptosis in the Failing Human Heart, *N. Engl. J. Med. 336*, 1131–1141.

57. Raff, M.C., Barres, B.A., Burne, J.F., Coles, H.S., Ishizaki, Y., and Jacobson, M.D. (1993) Programmed Cell Death and the Control of Cell Survival: Lessons from the Nervous System, *Science 262*, 695–700.

58. Mochizuki, H., Mori, H., and Mizuno, Y. (1997) Apoptosis in Neurodegenerative Disorders, *J. Neural. Transm. Suppl. 50*, 125–140.

59. Thompson, C.B. (1995) Apoptosis in the Pathogenesis and Treatment of Disease, *Science 267*, 1456–1462.

60. Yuan, J., Shaham, S., Ledoux, S., Ellis, H.M., and Horvitz, H.R. (1993) The *C. elegans* Cell Death Gene *ced-3* Encodes a Protein Similar to Mammalian Interleukin-1β Converting Enzyme, *Cell 75*, 641–752.

61. Hengartner, M.O., and Horvitz, H.R. (1994) *C. elegans* Cell Survival Gene ced-9 Encodes a Functional Homolog of the Mammalian Proto-Oncogene bcl-2, *Cell 76*, 665–676.

62. Pronk, G., Ramer, K., Amiri, P., and Williams, L. (1996) Requirement of an ICE-Like Protease for Induction of Apoptosis and Ceramide Generation by REAPER, *Science 271*, 808–810.

63. Yuan, J. (1996) Evolutionary Conservation of a Genetic Pathway of Programmed Cell Death, *J. Cell. Biochem. 60*, 4–11.

64. Lombardi, B., and Smith, M. L. (1994) Tumorigenesis, Protooncogene Activation, and Other Gene Abnormalities in Methyl Deficiency, *J. Nutr. Biochem. 5*, 2–9.

65. Albright, C.D., Lui, R., Bethea, T.C., da Costa, K.-A., Salganik, R.I., and Zeisel, S.H. (1996) Choline Deficiency Induces Apoptosis in SV40-Immortalized CWSV-1 Rat Hepatocytes in Culture, *FASEB J. 10*, 510–516.

66. Shin, O.H., Mar, M.H., Albright, C.D., Citarella, M.T., daCosta, K.A., and Zeisel, S.H. (1997) Methyl-Group Donors Cannot Prevent Apoptotic Death of Rat Hepatocytes Induced by Choline-Deficiency, *J. Cell. Biochem. 64*, 196–208.

67. Holmes-McNary, M.Q., Loy, R., Mar, M.-H., Albright, C.D., and Zeisel, S.H. (1997) Apoptosis is Induced by Choline Deficiency in Fetal Brain and in PC12 Cells, *Dev. Brain Res. 101*, 9–16.

68. Wolfe, J.T., Ross, D., and Cohen, G.M. (1994) A Role for Metals and Free Radicals in the Induction of Apoptosis in Thymocytes, *FEBS Lett. 352*, 58–62.

69. Slater, A.F., Nobel, C.S., and Orrenius, S. (1995) The Role of Intracellular Oxidants in Apoptosis, *Biochim. Biophys. Acta 1271*, 59–62.

70. Wood, K., and Youle, R. (1995) The Role of Free Radicals and p53 in Neuron Apoptosis In Vivo, *J. Neurosci. 15*, 5851–5857.

71. Kamata, H., Tanaka, C., Yagisawa, H., and Hirata, H. (1996) Nerve Growth Factor and Forskolin Prevent H_2O_2-Induced Apoptosis in PC12 Cells by Glutathione Independent Mechanism, *Neurosci. Lett. 212*, 179–182.

72. Hockenbery, D.M., Olivai, Z.N., Yin, X.M., Milliman, C.L., and Korsmeyer, S.J. (1993) Bcl-2 Functions in an Antioxidant Pathway to Prevent Apoptosis, *Cell 75*, 241–251.

73. Nakae, D., Yoshiji, H., Maruyama, H., Kinugasa, T., Denda, A., and Konishi, Y. (1990) Production of Both 8-Hydroxyguanosine in Liver DNA and γ-Glutamyltransferase-Positive Hepatocellular Lesions in Rats Given a Choline-Deficient, L-Amino Acid-Defined Diet, *Japan. J. Cancer Res. 81*, 1081–1084.

74. Haug, J.S., Goldner, C.M., Yazlovitskaya, E.M., Voziyan, P.A., and Melnykovych, G. (1994) Directed Cell Killing (Apoptosis) in Human Lymphoblastoid Cells Incubated in the Presence of Farnesol: Effect of Phosphatidylcholine, *Biochim. Biophys. Acta 1223*, 133–140.

75. Boggs, K.P., Rock, C.O., and Jackowski, S. (1995) Lysophosphatidylcholine Attenuates the Cytotoxic Effects of the Antineoplastic Phospholipid 1-O-octadecyl-2-O-methyl-*rac*-glycero-3-Phosphocholine, *J. Biol. Chem. 270*, 11612–11618.

76. Cui, Z., Houweling, M., Chen, M.H., Record, M., Chap, H., Vance, D.E., and Tercé, F. (1996) A Genetic Defect in Phosphatidylcholine Biosynthesis Triggers Apoptosis in Chinese Hamster Ovary Cells, *J. Biol. Chem. 271*, 14668–14671.

77. Jackowski, S. (1994) Coordination of Membrane Phospholipid Synthesis with the Cell Cycle, *J. Biol. Chem. 269*, 3858–3867.

78. Terce, F., Brun, H., and Vance, D.E. (1994) Requirement of Phosphatidylcholine for Normal Progression through the Cell Cycle in C3H/10T1/2 Fibroblasts, *J. Lipid Res. 35*, 2130–2142.

79. Verheij, M., Bose, R., Lin, X., Yao, B., Jarvis, W., Grant, S., Birrer, M., Szabo, E., and Kolesnick, R. (1996) Requirement for Ceramide-Initiated SAPK/JNK Signalling in Stress-Induced Apoptosis, *Nature 380*, 75–79.

80. Hartfield, P.J., Mayne, G.C., and Murray, A.W. (1997) Ceramide Induces Apoptosis in PC12 Cells, *FEBS Lett. 401*, 148–152.

81. Mizushima, N., Koike, R., Kohsaka, H., Kushi, Y., Handa, S., Yagita, H., and Miyasaka, N. (1996) Ceramide Induces Apoptosis via CPP32 Activation, *FEBS Lett. 395*, 267–271.

82. Toledano, B., Bastien, Y., Noya, F., Baruchel, S., and Mazer, B. (1997) Platelet-Activating Factor Abrogates Apoptosis Induced by Cross-Linking of the Surface IgM Receptor in a Human B Lymphoblastoid Cell Line, *J. Immunol. 158*, 3705–3715.

83. el Azzouzi, B., Jurgens, P., Benveniste, J., and Thomas, Y. (1993) Immunoregulatory Functions of PAF-Ac Ether. IX. Modulation of Apoptosis in an Immature T Cell Line, *Biochem. Biophys. Res. Commun. 190*, 320–324.

84. Cui, Z., and Vance, D.E. (1996) Expression of Phosphatidylethanolamine N-Methyltransferase-2 Is Markedly Enhanced in Long Term Choline-Deficient Rats, *J. Biol. Chem. 271*, 2839–2843.

85. Zeisel, S.H, daCosta, K.-A., Franklin, P.D., Alexander, E.A., Lamont, J.T., Sheard, N.F., and Beiser, A. (1991) Choline, an Essential Nutrient for Humans, *FASEB J. 5*, 2093–2098.

86. Buchman, A.L., Dubin, M., Jenden, D., Moukarzel, A., Roch, M.H., Rice, K., Gornbein, J., Ament, M.E., and Eckhert, C.D. (1992) Lecithin Increases Plasma Free Choline and Decreases Hepatic Steatosis in Long-Term Total Parenteral Nutrition Patients, *Gastroenterol. 102*, 1363–1370.

87. Buchman, A.L., Moukarzel, A., Jenden, D.J., Roch, M., Rice, K., and Ament, M.E. (1993) Low Plasma Free Choline Is Prevalent in Patients Receiving Long Term Parenteral Nutrition and Is Associated with Hepatic Aminotransferase Abnormalities, *Clin. Nutr. 12*, 33–37.

88. Buchman, A., Dubin, M., Moukarzel, A., Jenden, D., Roch, M., Rice, K., Gornbein, J., and Ament, M. (1995) Choline Deficiency: A Cause of Hepatic Steatosis During Parenteral Nutrition That Can Be Reversed with Intravenous Choline Supplementation, *Hepatol. 22*, 1399–1403.

89. Chandar, N., Amenta, J., Kandala, J.C., and Lombardi, B. (1987) Liver Cell Turnover in Rats Fed a Choline-Devoid Diet, *Carcinogenesis 8*, 669–673.

90. Christman, J.K., Chen, M. -L., Sheiknejad, G., Dizik, M., Abileah, S., and Wainfan, E. (1993) Methyl Deficiency, DNA Methylation and Cancer: Studies on the Reversibility of the Effects of a Lipotrope-Deficient Diet, *J. Nutr. Biochem. 4*, 672–680.

91. da Costa, K.-A., Garner, S.C., Chang, J., and Zeisel, S.H. (1995) Effects of Prolonged (I Year) Choline Deficiency and Subsequent Refeeding of Choline on 1,2-*sn*-Diradylglycerol, Fatty Acids and Protein Kinase C in Rat Liver, *Carcinogenesis 16*, 327–334.

92. da Costa, K., Cochary, E.F., Blusztajn, J.K., Garner, S.C., and Zeisel, S.H. (1993) Accumulation of 1,2-*sn*-Diradylglycerol with Increased Membrane-Associated Protein Kinase C May Be the Mechanism for Spontaneous Hepatocarcinogenesis in Choline Deficient Rats, *J. Biol. Chem. 268*, 2100–2105.

93. Ghoshal, A.K., Ahluwalia, M., and Farber, E. (1983) The Rapid Induction of Liver Cell Death in Rats Fed a Choline-Deficient Methionine-Low Diet, *Am. J. Pathol. 113*, 309–314.

94. Dizik, M., Christman, J.K., and Wainfan, E. (1991) Alterations in Expression and Methylation of Specific Genes in Livers of Rats Fed a Cancer Promoting Methyl-Deficient Diet, *Carcinogenesis 12*, 1307–1312.

95. Wainfan, E., and Poiner, L.A. (1992) Methyl Groups in Carcinogenesis: Effects on DNA Methylation and Gene Expression, *Cancer Res. 52*, 2071s–2077s.

96. Christman, J.K., Sheikhnejad, G., Dizik, M., Abileah, S., and Wainfan, E. (1993) Reversibility of Changes in Nucleic Acid Methylation and Gene Expression Induced in Rat Liver by Severe Dietary Methyl Deficiency, *Carcinogenesis 14*, 551–557.

97. Nakae, D., Yoshiji, H., Mizumoto, Y., Horiguchi, K., Shiraiwa, K., Tamura, K., Denda, A., and Konishi, Y. (1992) High Incidence of Hepatocellular Carcinomas Induced by a Choline Deficient L-Amino Acid Defined Diet in Rats, *Cancer Res. 52*, 5042–5045.

98. Nakae, D., Mizumoto, Y., Kobayashi, E., Noguchi, O., and Konishi, Y. (1995) Improved Genomic/Nuclear DNA Extraction for 8-Hydroxydeoxyguanosine Analysis of Small Amounts of Rat Liver Tissue, *Cancer Lett. 97*, 233–239.

Chapter 3

Phosphatidylethanolamine *N*-Methyltransferase: An Unexpected Regulator of Hepatocyte Cell Division

Dennis E. Vance[a], Zheng Cui[a], Martin Houweling[a], Christopher J. Walkey[a], and [b]Luciana Tessitore

[a]Lipid and Lipoprotein Research Group and Department of Biochemistry, University of Alberta, Edmonton, Alberta T6G 2S2, Canada, [b]Dipartimento di Scienze Cliniche e Biologiche, Università degli Studi di Torino, Torino, Italy

Phosphatidylcholine Biosynthesis

The major pathway for the biosynthesis of phosphatidylcholine (PC) in all mammalian nucleated cells is the cytidine diphosphate (CDP)–choline pathway. The rate-limiting and major regulatory reaction in the pathway is catalyzed by CTP:phosphocholine cytidylyltransferase (CT) (1). A second pathway found in mammalian cells is the reacylation of lyso-PC, which can be supplied to cells by serum or be derived in cells by deacylation of PC. The quantitative significance of the reacylation pathway in PC biosynthesis is unknown. A third pathway is the conversion of phosphatidylethanolamine (PE) to PC, catalyzed by phosphatidylethanolamine *N*-methyltransferase (PEMT). This reaction occurs primarily in hepatocytes; it is present at 2% or less in nonhepatic cells (2). Thus, the methylation of PE is of quantitative significance only in hepatocytes.

The activity of CT is regulated by translocation from a soluble form, which is inactive, to a membrane-bound form, which is active (1). An increase in activity of CT is promoted by a decrease in cellular PC, an increase in the supply of fatty acids to the cell, or an increase in diacylglycerol (1); a decrease in CT activity occurs under opposite conditions, such as an abundance of PC. Both forms of the enzyme are localized to the nucleus in CHO (Chinese hamster ovary) cells and in some other dividing cells (3), whereas in primary rat hepatocytes, which do not divide, CT is largely found outside of the nucleus (4). CT has been purified to homogeneity from rat liver (5) and the cDNA cloned from a rat liver library and expressed (6). A partial sequence of the CT gene has been reported and the gene localized to chromosome 16 on the mouse genome (7). Transgenic expression of CT in mice has not been reported.

PEMT was purified to homogeneity in 1987 (8) and the cDNA cloned and expressed (9). A peptide was synthesized according to the sequence of the carboxyl terminus, and a polyclonal antibody to that peptide was prepared and used in immunoblot studies on subcellular fractions of rat liver. Surprisingly, the antibody was found to cross-react only with a protein from the mitochondria-associated membrane, a subsection of the endoplasmic reticulum that fractionates with mitochondria after homogenization and centrifugation (9,10). There was no reaction with proteins from the endoplasmic reticulum, even though 70–80% of PEMT activity in liver resides in this fraction (9). Hence, the cloned cDNA appears to code for a previously unknown form of the enzyme, now referred to as PEMT2. The activity on the endoplasmic reticulum is referred to as PEMT1.

The murine gene for PEMT2 has recently been cloned and characterized (11). In mice, PEMT2 arises from a single-copy gene that spans at least 35 kb, with seven exons and six introns, located on chromosome 11. A targeting vector for disruption of the PEMT2 gene in mice has been constructed and heterozygous mice obtained in which one copy of the gene has been disrupted (Walkey, C.J., and Vance, D.E., unpublished results). These mice will be bred to obtain homozygous mice in which both copies of the gene have been disrupted. Those mice should provide unique information about the function of PEMT2 in control of hepatocyte cell division and its potential role as a tumor suppressor, as discussed in subsequent sections.

PC Biosynthesis and Cell Division

Since PC is the major membrane phospholipid in most eukaryotic cells, it is not surprising that the biosynthesis of PC is an important and critical reaction for eukaryotic cell division (PC is absent from almost all prokaryotes). A large increase in the biosynthesis of PC and other phospholipids is required for the doubling of the cell components that occurs at each cell division. Increased phospholipid biosynthesis occurs during S phase after transition from G0 to G1 (12,13). Recently, in a macrophage cell line, PC was shown to accumulate during the S phase of the cell cycle, and CT activity was maximal during G1 (14).

Choline, the precursor for PC, is absolutely required for growth of cultured cells (15) and is an essential nutrient for mammals (16). We recently demonstrated, using choline deficiency as a model system, that PC biosynthesis was required for normal progression through the cell cycle in fibroblasts (17). Of the cells that were deprived of choline, 85% accumulated in the G1 phase of cell division. When these choline-deficient cells were supplemented with choline, synchronous cell division occurred (17). Thus, it appears that PC biosynthesis is required for normal progression beyond the G1 phase of the cell cycle.

The importance of PC biosynthesis for cell division was strikingly demonstrated by the isolation of temperature-sensitive mutants of CHO cells in which CT was inactivated at the restrictive temperature of 40°C; the cells died (18). We were curious as to whether PC biosynthesis *via* the CDP-choline pathway was required for cell division and whether the PEMT2 pathway could replace the CDP-choline pathway. Thus, we took advantage of this CHO cell line with a temperature-sensitive defect in CT. The mutant CHO cells were transfected with PEMT2 behind the cytomegalovirus promoter, and stable cell lines were isolated (19). Suprisingly, although the transfected cells restored the normal level of PC *via* the methylation of PE, these cells still did not survive at the restrictive temperature of 40°C. Thus, the data clearly showed that methylation of PE to PC could not substitute for the CDP-choline pathway in these cells.

It was surprising that a cell with defective synthesis of PC would die immediately rather than remain quiescent, as might be observed with nutrient deprivation. An answer to this curiosity came from the discovery that a sudden cascade of apoptosis was triggered in the mutant immediately after the complete shutdown of the CDP-choline pathway at the restrictive temperature (20). Additionally, this activation of cell suicide appears specific to the CDP-choline pathway, because the functional expression of PEMT2 failed to rescue the mutant at the restrictive temperature. These results agree with the finding that immortalized CWSV-1 rat hepatocytes also undergo apoptosis when choline is removed from the medium (21). We have also shown that rat hepatoma cells die, probably *via* apoptosis, when deprived of choline for more than 24 h.

Taken together, the data provide a strong case for the CDP-choline pathway having an intimate relationship with at least one apoptotic pathway in mammalian cells, in addition to its strong association with cellular proliferation. Furthermore, the unique function of the CDP-choline pathway cannot be replaced by the PE methylation pathway. If the function of the PE methylation pathway is not to replace or back up the CDP-choline pathway, why does liver still possess this ancient PE methyltransferase, which can be traced back in evolution as far as *Rhodobacteria* and yeast?

A Role for PEMT2 in Regulation of Hepatocyte Cell Division

Whereas primary liver hepatocytes express approximately 1 nmol/min/mg of protein of PEMT activity, McArdle cells have only 20 pmol/min/mg protein of PEMT activity (22). We were curious as to what would happen to the CDP-choline pathway in McArdle cells if we overexpressed PEMT2. Therefore, McArdle RH7777 hepatoma cells were transfected with PEMT2 behind the cytomegalovirus promoter, and stable cell lines were obtained (22). Surprisingly, in the course of these experiments we observed that the rate of cell division was slowed in the PEMT2-transfected cells. There was a linear correlation between the time for cell division and the extent of PEMT2 expression. Normally, McArdle cells require 18 to 20 h for a cell cycle, but cells that expressed over 600 pmol/min/mg protein of PEMT2 activity required approximately 50 h to complete a cycle of cell division (22). Numerous control experiments showed that the effect on cell division was not an artifact. These experiments clearly demonstrated an unexpected role for PEMT2 in the control of hepatoma cell division.

Next, we studied the effect of PEMT2 overexpression on CT and the CDP-choline pathway. The results showed that as the expression of PEMT2 increased, there was a concomitant decrease in CT expression in the McArdle hepatoma cells (23). The changes occurred at the level of gene expression, since the mRNA for CT was decreased, as determined by Northern blots, as was the amount of CT protein detected by immunoblot analyses. Thus, one possibility is that the observed effect of

PEMT2 on hepatoma cell division could be related to the down-regulation of CT and the CDP-choline pathway.

The studies with PEMT2-transfected hepatoma cells strongly suggested an unexpected role for this enzyme in the regulation of normal hepatocyte cell division. Subsequently, we have extended these studies to three models in intact rats in which hepatocytes have been induced to divide.

In the first model, we subjected adult rats to partial hepatectomy. In this procedure, approximately 2/3 of the liver is surgically removed; the liver subsequently regenerates over a period of one week, involving many divisions of the remaining hepatocytes. At various times after the procedure, we measured the activities, the amount of protein, and the levels of mRNA for PEMT2 and CT. The activity of PEMT (measuring both PEMT1 and PEMT2) was decreased by 50% at 24 h after the operation and gradually returned to normal levels 192 h after the operation (24). The results with PEMT2 were more striking. After 24 h, the protein and mRNA for this enzyme had almost completely disappeared. The levels were restored to normal amounts after 192 h. In contrast, the activity of CT, the amount of CT protein, and the CT mRNA were all elevated approximately twofold 24 h after partial hepatectomy and gradually returned to preoperation levels during the next 7 d. These data provided the first *in vivo* relationships among hepatocyte cell division, decrease in PEMT2 expression, and increase in CT expression.

The second model consisted of investigating the expression of PEMT2 and CT as a function of development of rat liver. The liver grows rapidly during days 17 to 21 of gestation; at birth the rate of liver growth slows significantly. Thirty-five days after birth, the rat liver is fully mature. Once again there was an inverse correlation between the rate of hepatocyte cell division and the expression of PEMT2. Before birth, PEMT2 was not expressed (25). At birth, PEMT2 was induced to 50% of its adult value, as assessed by measuring mRNA and immunoblots. The expression of PEMT2 gradually increased during the next 21 d to adult values. In contrast, CT activity was at its highest level 5 d before birth and gradually decreased during development to its adult values. Thus, the inverse correlation between hepatocyte cell division and PEMT2 activity was observed again during development of the rat liver. In contrast, there was a good correlation between the rate of hepatocyte cell division and CT activity.

The third model consisted of inducing hepatocyte proliferation by injection of mature animals with lead nitrate. Once again, we observed a good correlation between hepatocyte cell division and CT activity and an inverse correlation between hepatocyte cell division and PEMT2 expression (26).

When the foregoing cell culture and *in vivo* studies are considered together, there is a strong case for a role for PEMT2 in the regulation of hepatocyte cell division. It is of great interest whether or not the lipid product of PE methylation controls liver proliferation directly or indirectly via other cellular processes. PEMT2 is probably only one of many players that might coordinate a hepatocyte's preparations for cell division. One of our hypotheses is that PEMT2 regulates the supply of PC for the process of cell division. The present evidence suggests that PEMT2 may achieve this function by control of CT activity. The role for PEMT2 in control of cell division appears to be restricted to hepatocytes, because they are the only cells in which it is expressed (9). Moreover, expression of PEMT2 in CHO cells had no effect on cell division or on the expression of CT (19, 27).

PEMT2—A Candidate Tumor Suppressor

As already discussed, when we transfected McArdle RH7777 hepatoma cells with PEMT2 behind the cytomegalovirus promoter, stable cell lines were obtained (22). In these cells there was a linear correlation between the time for cell division and the extent of PEMT2 expression: McArdle cells require 18 to 20 h for a cell cycle, whereas cells transfected with PEMT2 required approximately 50 h to complete cell division (22). Because of this observation, we did a preliminary experiment on the expression of PEMT2 in carcinogen-induced rat liver cancer. The results showed an almost complete disappearance of PEMT2 in cancer nodules compared to normal liver (22). A more complete study has now shown that PEMT2 is inactivated in rat liver tumors and precancerous lesions induced by treatment with diethylnitrosamine or methylnitrosourea (26). Expression of PEMT2 was decreased by 60% in liver samples with the first detectable proliferative nodules. By the time the cancer reached the hepatoma stage, there was no expression of PEMT2. At the hepatoma stage of liver carcinogenesis, there was an induction of CT.

Therefore, the following facts suggest that PEMT2 might be considered an unusual tumor suppressor:

1. PEMT2 is present only in trace amounts in human and rat hepatoma cell lines (human HepG2 and rat McArdle RH7777 cells), whereas PEMT2 is abundantly expressed in normal hepatocytes (22).

2. A cause-and-effect relationship is established, because expression of PEMT2, but not other proteins, in McArdle cells increases the time required for cell division threefold (22).

3. PEMT2 expression is decreased at the earliest stages of hepatocarcinogenesis induced by diethylnitrosamine or methylnitrosourea.

Experiments are currently underway to determine by Southern blot analyses whether or not the PEMT2 gene is intact in the carcinogen-treated rat livers. Whatever the result, some role for PEMT2 in certain forms of liver carcinogenesis seems very likely.

Conclusion

For decades it has been clear that PC biosynthesis has an important role in eukaryotic cells. Clearly, supply of the main phospholipid of cellular membranes is a key, fundamental role. However, work in the last few years has revealed the unexpected finding that CT and the CDP-choline pathway have a role in cell division beyond providing a major component of membranes. Exactly what this role is remains to be determined. Why PEMT2 will not satisfy the need of cells in culture for CT and the CDP-choline pathway is also unexplained.

Why has it evolved that PEMT2 has such an apparently important role in control of hepatocyte cell division? Is PEMT2 essential, or can some other enzyme such as PEMT1 take its place? The answer to this question should be forthcoming after homozygous mice are obtained in which the PEMT2 gene has been disrupted.

Finally, at this stage there are intriguing indications that PEMT2 might have a tumor suppressor role. Whether this is true in human primary liver cancer needs to be investigated.

References

1. Vance, D.E. (1996) in *Biochemistry of Lipids, Lipoproteins and Membranes,* Vance, D.E. and Vance, J.E., eds., Elsevier, Amsterdam, pp. 153–181.

2. Vance, D.E., and Ridgway, N.D. (1988) The Methylation of Phosphatidylethanol-amine, *Prog. Lipid Res. 27,* 61–79.

3. Kent, C. (1995) Eukaryotic Phospholipid Biosynthesis, *Annu. Rev. Biochem. 64,* 315–343.

4. Houweling, M., Cui, Z., Anfuso, C.D., Bussière, M., Chen, M.H., and Vance, D.E. (1996) CTP:Phosphocholine Cytidylyltransferase Is Both a Nuclear and Cytoplasmic Protein in Primary Hepatocytes, *Europ. J. Cell Biol. 69,* 55–63.

5. Feldman, D.A., and Weinhold, P.A. (1987) CTP:Phosphorylcholine Cytidylyltransferase from Rat Liver: Isolation and Characterization of the Catalytic Subunit, *J. Biol. Chem. 262,* 9075–9081.

6. Kalmar, G.B., Kay, R.J., Lachance, A., Aebersold, R., and Cornell, R.B. (1990) Cloning and Expression of Rat Liver CTP:Phosphocholine Cytidylyltransferase: An Amphipathic Protein That Controls Phosphatidylcholine Synthesis, *Proc. Natl. Acad. Sci. USA 87,* 6029–6033.

7. Rutherford, M.S., Rock, C.O., Jenkins, N.A., Gilbert, D.J., Tessner, T.G., Copeland, N.G., and Jackowski, S. (1993) The Gene for Murine CTP:Phosphocholine Cytidylyltransferase (Cptct) Is Located on Mouse Chromosome 16, *Genomics 18,* 698–701.

8. Ridgway, N.D., and Vance, D.E. (1987) Purification of Phosphatidylethanolamine *N*-Methyltransferase from Rat Liver, *J. Biol. Chem. 262,* 17231–17239.

9. Cui, Z., Vance, J.E., Chen, M.H., Voelker, D.R., and Vance, D.E. (1993) Cloning and Expression of a Novel Phosphatidylethanolamine *N*-Methyltransferase, *J. Biol. Chem. 268,* 16655–16663.

10. Vance, J.E. (1990) Phospholipid Synthesis in a Membrane Fraction Associated with Mitochondria, *J. Biol. Chem. 265,* 7248–7256.

11. Walkey, C.J., Cui, Z., Agellon, L.B., and Vance, D.E. (1996) Characterization of the Murine Phosphatidylethanolamine *N*-Methyltransferase-2 Gene, *J. Lipid Res.,* in press.

12. Cunningham, D.D., and Pardee, A.B. (1969) Transport Changes Rapidly Initiated by Serum Addition to "Contact Inhibited" 3T3 Cells, *Biochemistry 64,* 1049–1056.

13. Bergeron, J.J.M., Warmsley, A.M.H., and Pasternak, C.A. (1970) Phospholipid Synthesis and Degradation During the Life-Cycle of P815Y Mast Cells Synchronized with Excess of Thymidine, *Biochem. J. 119,* 489–492.

14. Jackowski, S. (1994) Coordination of Membrane Phospholipid Synthesis with the Cell Cycle, *J. Biol. Chem. 269,* 3858–3867.

15. Eagle, H. (1955) The Minimum Vitamin Requirements of the L and HeLa Cells in Tissue Culture, the Production of Specific Vitamin Deficiencies, and Their Cure, *J. Exp. Med. 102,* 595–600.

16. Zeisel, S.H., and Blusztajn, J.K. (1994) Choline and Human Nutrition, *Annu. Rev. Nutr. 14,* 269–296.

17. Tercé, R., Brun, H., and Vance, D.E. (1994) Requirement of Phosphatidylcholine for Normal Progression Through the Cell Cycle in C3H/10T1/2 Fibroblasts, *J. Lipid Res. 35,* 2130–2142.

18. Esko, J.D., Wermuth, M.M., and Raetz, C.H.R. (1981) Thermolabile CDP-Choline Synthetase in an Animal Cell Mutant Defective in Lecithin Formation, *J. Biol. Chem. 256,* 7388–7393.

19. Houweling, M., Cui, Z., and Vance, D.E. (1995) Expression of Phosphatidylethanolamine *N*-Methyltransferase-2 Cannot Compensate for an Impaired CDP-Choline Pathway in Mutant Chinese Hamster Ovary Cells, *J. Biol. Chem. 270,* 16277–16282.

20. Cui, Z., Houweling, M., Chen, M.H., Record, M., Chap, H., Vance, D.E., and Tercé, F. (1996) A Genetic Defect in Phosphatidylcholine Biosynthesis Triggers Apoptosis in Chinese Hamster Ovary Cells, *J. Biol. Chem. 271,* 14668–14671.

21. Albright, C.D., Liu, R., Bethea, T.C., da Costa, K.-A., Salganik, R.I., and Zeisel, S.H. (1996) Choline Deficiency Induces Apoptosis in SV40-Immortalized CWSV-1 Rat Hepatocytes in Culture, *FASEB J. 10,* 510–516.

22. Cui, Z., Houweling, M., and Vance, D.E. (1994) Suppression of Rat Hepatoma Cell Growth by Expression of Phosphatidylethanolamine *N*-Methyltransferase-2, *J. Biol. Chem. 269,* 24531–24533.

23. Cui, Z., Houweling, M., and Vance, D.E. (1995) Expression of Phosphatidylethanolamine *N*-Methyltransferase-2 in McArdle-RH7777 Hepatoma Cells Inhibits the CDP-Choline Pathway for Phosphatidylcholine Biosynthesis via Decreased Gene Expression of CTP:Phosphocholine Cytidylyltransferase, *Biochem. J. 312,* 939–945.

24. Houweling, M., Cui, Z., Tessitore, L., and Vance, D.D. (1997) Induction of Hepatocyte Proliferation After Partial Hepatectomy Is Accompanied by a Markedly Reduced Expression of Phosphatidylethanolamine *N*-Methyltransferase-2, *Biochim. Biophys. Acta 1346,* 1–9.

25. Cui, Z., Shen, Y.-J., and Vance, D.E. (1997) Inverse Correlation Between Expression of Phosphatidylethanolamine *N*-Methyltransferase-2 and the Growth Rate of Perinatal Rat Livers, *Biochim. Biophys. Acta 1346,* 10–16.

26. Tessitore, L., Cui, Z., and Vance, D.E. (1997) Transient Inactivation of Phosphatidylethanolamine *N*-Methyltransferase-2 and Activation of Cytidine Triphosphate:Phosphocholine Cytidyltransferase During Non-Neoplastic Liver Growth, *Biochem. J. 322,* 151–154.

27. Lee, M.W., Bakovic, M., and Vance, D.E. (1996) Overexpression of Phosphatidylethanolamine Methyltransferase-2 (PEMT2) in CHO-K1 Cells Does Not Attenuate the Activity of the CDP-Choline Pathway for Phosphatidylcholine Biosynthesis, *Biochem. J. 320,* 905–910.

Chapter 4

Antineoplastic Phospholipids Inhibit Phosphatidylcholine Biosynthesis

Suzanne Jackowski[a] and Kevin Boggs[b]

[a]Department of Biochemistry, St. Jude Children's Research Hospital, Memphis, TN 38101,
Department of Biochemistry, University of Tennessee, Memphis, TN 38163,
[b]Department of Biochemistry, St. Jude Children's Research Hospital, Memphis, TN 38101

Antineoplastic Phospholipids

Interest in ether-linked phospholipid analogs as antineoplastic compounds is growing, because they do not directly target DNA and could potentially complement existing DNA-directed anticancer compounds. A comparison of the structures of these phospholipid analogs to lysophosphatidylcholine (LPC) is shown in Fig. 4.1. All of the active compounds have a choline group attached to a hydrocarbon tail that mimics the extended configuration of LPC. Stereochemistry is not a critical feature of the molecules. Some compounds, such as hexadecylphosphocholine (HexPC), do not have a chiral center; both stereoisomers of 1-*O*-octadecyl-2-*O*-methyl-*rac*-glycero-3-phosphocholine (ET-18-OCH$_3$) are cytotoxic toward HL-60 cells (1). Numerous studies have demonstrated the selective cytotoxic action of ET-18-OCH$_3$ against transformed cells in whole animals and tissue culture (2–11). Ongoing clinical trials are evaluating the effectiveness of different antineoplastic ether-linked phospholipid analogs against a variety of cancers; for review, see Ref. 12. One example of clinical research is the use of ET-18-OCH$_3$ to purge leukemic bone marrow for autologous bone marrow transplantation (13,14).

Many biological processes have been suggested as primary targets for ET-18-OCH$_3$ action; for review, see Ref. 15.

- ET-18-OCH$_3$ has detergent properties, spontaneously transfers between membrane systems (8), and will lyse cells at high concentrations (16). However, the detergent action of the compound does not account for its biological activity, because cell growth is inhibited at low concentrations of ET-18-OCH$_3$, and exposure of cells to the same concentrations of similar detergents such as LPC does not affect proliferation.

- ET-18-OCH$_3$ also does not function as an analog of platelet-activating factor (17–19).

- Protein kinase C is a definitive target for ET-18-OCH$_3$ inhibition *in vitro* (for review, see Ref. 15), and several protein kinase C–regulated functions are blocked by ET-18-OCH$_3$ *in vivo* (20.21). However, recent data argue against

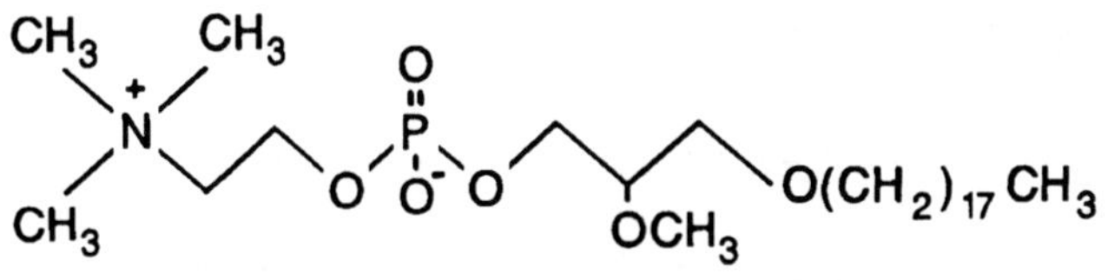

ET-18-OCH$_3$ (Edelfosine)

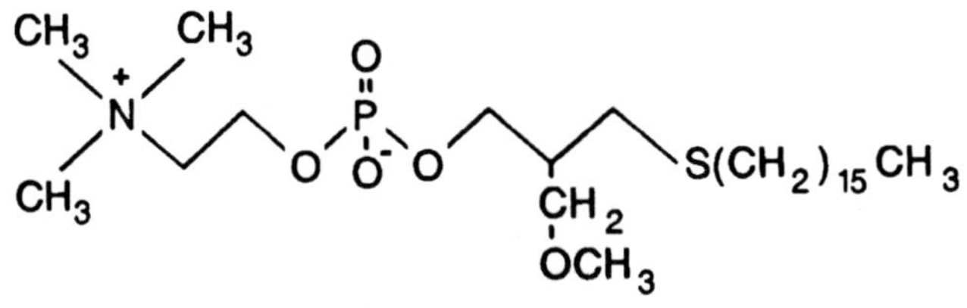

BM 41.440 (Ilmofosine)

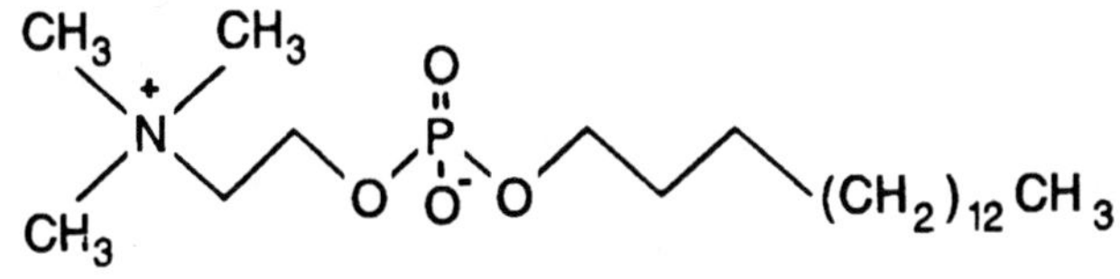

HexPC (Miltefosine)

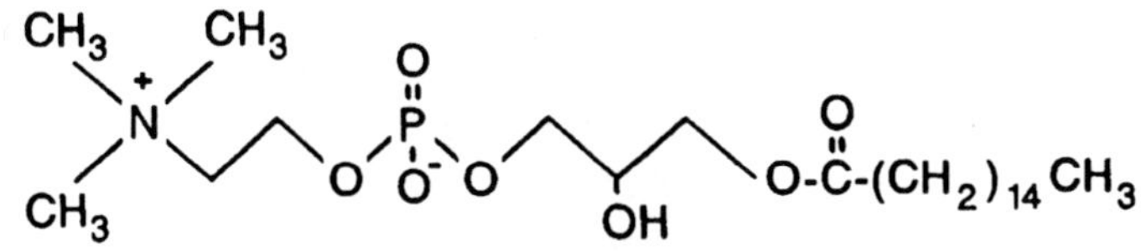

LPC (1-Acyl-GPC)

Fig. 4.1. Structures of three representative antineoplastic lipids. The principal ether lipid that is discussed is 1-*O*-octadecyl-2-*O*-methyl-*rac*-glycero-3-phosphocholine (ET-18-OCH₃, edelfosine). A variety of modifications at the 2-position illustrate that the methoxy group is not essential; one of these biologically active derivatives is BM 41.440 (ilmofosine). The glycerol backbone can also be eliminated with retention of biological activity; hexadecyl-phosphocholine (HexPC, mitelfosine) is an example. These drugs are structural analogs of lysophosphatidylcholine (LPC).

protein kinase C as an intracellular target relevant to cellular growth control by antineoplastic phospholipid analogs (22,23).

- ET-18-OCH$_3$ blocks the hydrolysis of polyphosphoinositides that is initiated by platelet-derived growth factor (PDGF) receptor stimulation, and blocks the activity of phospholipases Cγ and δ *in vitro* (24–26). However, the concentrations of ET-18-OCH$_3$ required to block phospholipase Cγ or δ calcium mobilization are 10 times higher than the concentrations required to block cell growth, suggesting that these phospholipases are not the most important targets.

The hypothesis that will be explored in this review is that the inhibition of membrane phospholipid formation by antineoplastic phospholipids triggers apoptosis and accounts for their cytotoxicity.

CT Is a Key Regulator of Phospholipid Synthesis

CTP:phosphocholine cytidylyltransferase (CT) is the rate-controlling enzyme for PtdCho biosynthesis in mammalian cells (Fig. 4.2) (27–29) and is therefore likely to play a role in the inhibition of PtdCho synthesis by antineoplastic phospholipids. CT activity is necessary for cell survival in cultured eukaryotic cells (30), not only because PtdCho is the major membrane constituent but also because it is a precursor to the two other most abundant membrane phospholipids: sphingomyelin (31) and phosphatidylethanolamine (32).

   Distinct domains in CT are responsible for the positive regulation of activity by lipid modulators or negative regulation by phosphorylation (Fig. 4.3). CT exhibits negligible activity *in vitro* in the absence of lipid activators, and its potent stimulation by lipids is thought to make a significant contribution to controlling the activity of the enzyme *in vivo*. CT activity is stimulated by acidic lipids (such as oleic acid) or diacylglycerol incorporated into PtdCho bilayers (33–35). Accordingly, addition of exogenous oleic acid and addition of PtdCho-specific phospholipase C (to generate cellular DAG) are both associated with enhanced rates of PtdCho synthesis and increased association of CT with cellular membranes (36–40). CT activity and membrane association increase in cells deficient in PtdCho, correlating with the increased relative abundance of anionic phospholipids (41–44). Kinetic analysis of CT in the presence and absence of lipid activators shows that activating lipids increase CT activity by increasing the affinity of the protein for the nucleotide CTP (45). Analysis of the predicted amino acid sequence derived from rat CT cDNA shows a region between residues 251 and 286 of the protein that constitutes an amphipathic helical domain similar to lipoprotein domains known to interact directly with phospholipids (46); see Fig. 4.3. Evidence obtained from limited chymotrypsin proteolysis (47), from deletion mutagenesis, (45,48) and by using antibodies directed against the helical region (49) is consistent with the idea that the helical domain is responsible for the lipid regulation of CT activity.

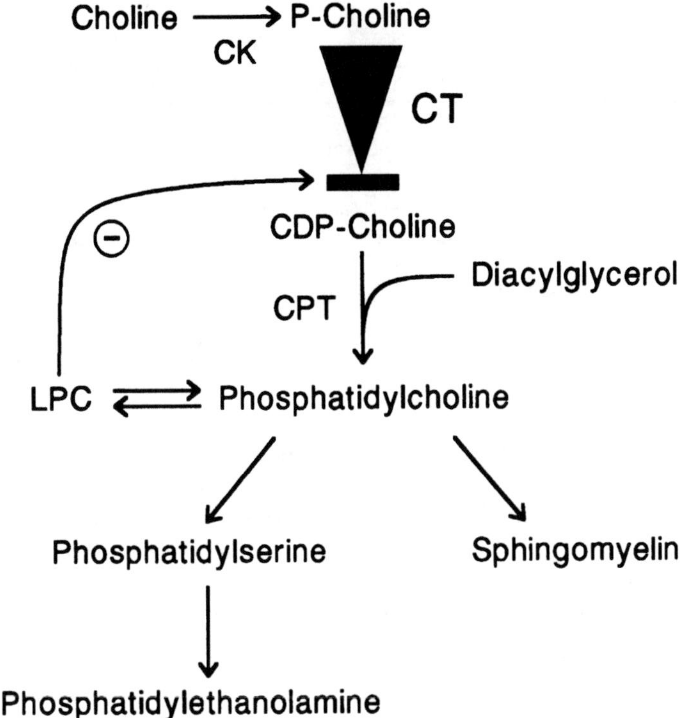

Fig. 4.2. Pathways for membrane phospholipid synthesis. The synthesis of PtdCho begins with the transport of choline into the cell and its phosphorylation by choline kinase (CK). CT catalyzes the rate-controlling step in the pathway, and the CDP-choline formed in this reaction is converted to PtdCho by choline phosphotransferase (CPT). LPC is a physiological inhibitor of *de novo* PtdCho biosynthesis at the CT step. The antineoplastic phospholipids ET-18-OCH$_3$ and HexPC are nonmetabolizable analogs of LPC that are proposed to inhibit membrane phospholipid formation at the CT step by mimicking the action of LPC. (*Source:* Boggs, K.P., et al. (1995) *J. Biol. Chem. 270*, 7757–7764. Reprinted with permission.)

CT is extensively phosphorylated at multiple sites *in vivo*. Detailed analysis of CT phosphorylation shows that these sites are exclusively located in the carboxy terminal domain (residues 312–367) of the protein (50); see Fig. 4.3. Experiments with purified CT and CT mutants establish that phosphorylation inhibits CT activity by negatively regulating the binding of CT to lipid activators (51). The correlations between the degree of CT phosphorylation and the activity and membrane association of CT in Chinese hamster ovary (52) and HeLa cells (53),

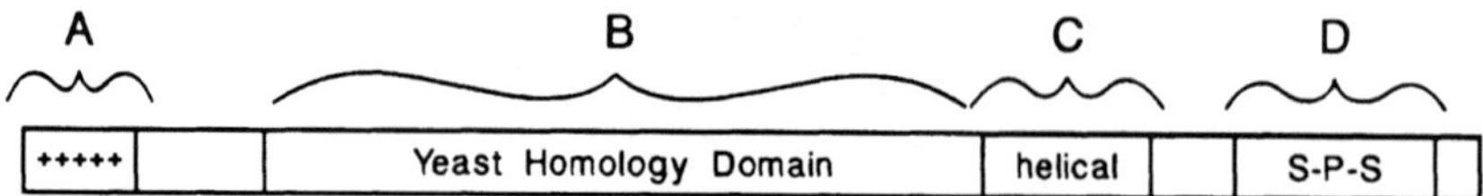

Fig. 4.3. Domain structure of CT. The primary sequence of CT is divided into four functional domains: A, a cluster of positively charged amino acids at the amino terminus that functions as a nuclear localization signal; B, the yeast homology domain—that is, the active site of the protein, where CTP and phosphocholine bind; C, the helical region, composed of three consecutive amphipathic helices that are responsible for the activation of the enzyme *via* their interaction with activating lipid embedded in the membrane bilayer; D, the carboxy-terminal Ser/Pro-rich region that contains all of the known phosphorylation sites on the protein.

the stimulation of PtdCho synthesis by exogenous oleic acid (53), and the decrease in PtdCho synthesis in cells treated with the phosphatase inhibitor okadaic acid (54) are all consistent with this idea. However, the pattern of CT phosphorylation *in vivo* is complex (50,52,55–57). The negative correlation between CT phosphorylation and membrane association is not always observed (57), indicating that carboxy terminal phosphorylation modifies the affinity of CT for membranes but probably cannot completely prevent CT binding to membranes that contain high concentrations of activating lipids.

LPC Regulates PtdCho Synthesis at the CT Step

We have investigated the regulation of the CDP-choline pathway of PtdCho synthesis at the CT step by LPC in a colony-stimulating factor 1 (CSF-1)-dependent murine macrophage cell line (58). LPC strongly inhibited phosphatidylcholine synthesis *in vivo* (Fig. 4.4) and led to the accumulation of choline and phosphocholine along with the disappearance of CDP-choline. These data point to CT as the intracellular target. LPC neither inhibited cell growth, decreased the cellular content of CT, nor altered the distribution of CT between soluble and particulate subcellular fractions. The inhibition of phosphatidylcholine synthesis was specific to LPC; lysophospholipids that lacked the choline headgroup were not inhibitors. LPC inhibited CT activity *in vitro*; kinetic analysis showed that the inhibition was competitive with respect to the lipid activator. The physiological significance of these observations can be understood according to the model shown in Fig. 4.2. Exogenous LPC is converted directly to PtdCho by LPC acyltransferase (59), therefore obviating the need for PtdCho production via the CDP-choline pathway. Thus, LPC acts as a negative physiological regulator of PtdCho synthesis by inhibiting the *de novo* pathway at the CT step and at the same time can bypass the biosynthetic block.

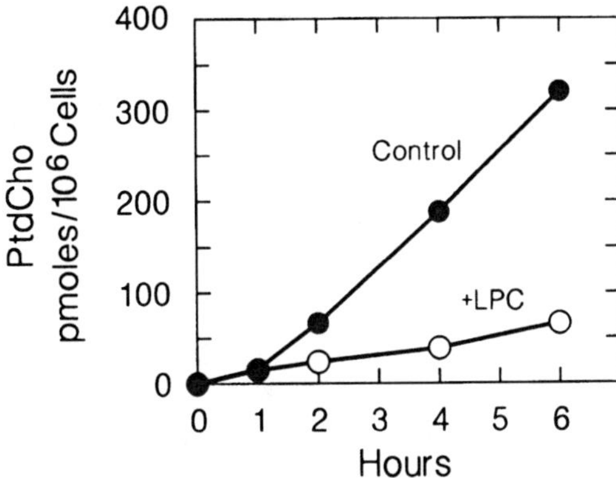

Fig. 4.4. Inhibition of PtdCho synthesis by LPC. A time course for [³H]choline uptake into the PtdCho fraction of BAC1.2F5 cells in the presence and absence of 200 µM LPC. (*Source:* Boggs, K.P., et al. (1995) *J. Biol. Chem. 270*, 7757–7764. Reprinted with permission.)

Antineoplastic Phospholipids Inhibit PtdCho Synthesis at the CT Step

In 1979, Modolell et al. (60) reported that ET-18-OCH$_3$-treated cells had reduced levels of PtdCho. Subsequently, several groups showed that ET-18-OCH$_3$ decreases choline incorporation into PtdCho (61–64). The mechanism for inhibition of this pathway was not established, although ET-18-OCH$_3$ was reported to diminish the association of CT with the membrane (64). A related analog, HexPC, also inhibited choline incorporation into PtdCho (65–67) and partially inhibited CT activity when added to whole-cell lysates (68). Our group investigated the interference of antineoplastic phospholipids with PtdCho synthesis in a macrophage cell line (58,69) and HL-60 cells (see below). Our results strongly support the idea that inhibition of PtdCho synthesis is responsible for the cytotoxic action of antineoplastic phospholipids. We have confirmed that ET-18-OCH$_3$ is a potent inhibitor of PtdCho synthesis in our BAC1.2F5 macrophage cell line and the pattern of accumulation of soluble intermediates within the first 2 h of labeling point to CT as the inhibited step *in vivo* (58). Confirmation that CT was a relevant target came from analysis of the inhibition of CT activity *in vitro* by ET-18-OCH$_3$ (Fig. 4.5). As with LPC, ET-18-OCH$_3$ inhibition of CT was competitive with respect to lipid activator. The inhibition of CT by LPC and ET-18-OCH$_3$ is reminiscent of the negative regulation of this enzyme by sphingosine (70).

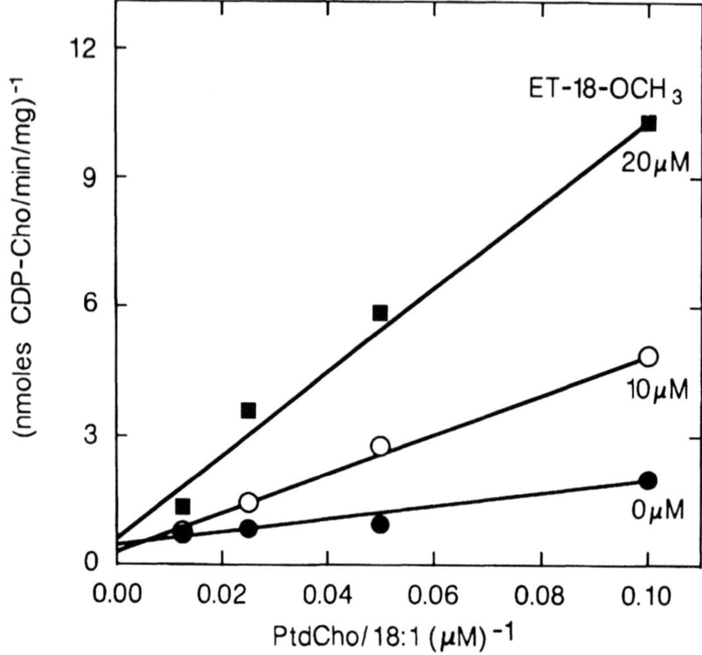

Fig. 4.5. Competitive inhibition of CT activity by ET-18-OCH$_3$. CT was purified and assayed in the presence of the indicated concentrations of lipid activators and ET-18-OCH$_3$. The results, displayed as a double-reciprocal plot, indicate that ET-18-OCH$_3$ is a competitive inhibitor with respect to the lipid activator. (*Source:* Boggs, K.P., et al. (1995) *J. Biol. Chem. 270*, 7757–7764. Reprinted with permission.)

Antineoplastic Phospholipids Induce Apoptosis

The cell death triggered by ET-18-OCH$_3$ and other antineoplastic phospholipids has been established to result from apoptosis (69,71–73). ET-18-OCH$_3$-treated cells exhibit all of the hallmark features of apoptosis, including cell shrinkage, nuclear condensation, and DNA fragmentation. The morphological features of apoptosis are clearly evident in the BAC1.2F5 macrophage cell line treated with ET-18-OCH$_3$ (Fig. 4.6, panels B and C). The importance of these observations is that they establish that ET-18-OCH$_3$ inhibits a physiological process, triggering the cells to undergo a program of cell death.

LPC Prevents ET-18-OCH$_3$-Induced Apoptosis

LPC circumvents the requirement for *de novo* PtdCho biosynthesis via the CDP-choline pathway (74), and LPC analogs strongly inhibit choline incorporation into loss of phospholipid asymmetry, even though the distribution of only one lipid species—PS—is being measured. It is also often assumed that PS is reaching the surface from the inner leaflet of the plasma membrane and not by some other mechanism, such as addition of new membrane to the plasma membrane during exocytosis.

While these assays are invaluable in establishing the equilibrium distribution of phospholipids, insight into how these distributions come about and their underlying dynamics has come from assays that measure transbilayer movement of phospholipids. Such assays reveal the existence of two membrane activities that govern the distribution of phospholipids and that also serve to illustrate the assays that detect them.

The Aminophospholipid Translocase

Because phospholipids diffuse passively across biological membranes over the course of several hours, the persistence of a nonrandom distribution of phospholipids immediately implies an active process at work. In fact, the plasma membranes of every cell thus far examined, from erythrocytes to fibroblasts to sperm, and the membranes of some internal transport vesicles as well, all contain an ATP-dependent activity that specifically transports aminophospholipids from the extracytosolic to the cytosolic side of the membrane (Fig. 6.1).

This translocase activity is revealed in assays of transbilayer lipid movement such as the one presented in Fig. 6.2. Fluorescent phospholipid analogs were introduced into the outer leaflet of the plasma membrane of *T* lymphocyte hybridoma

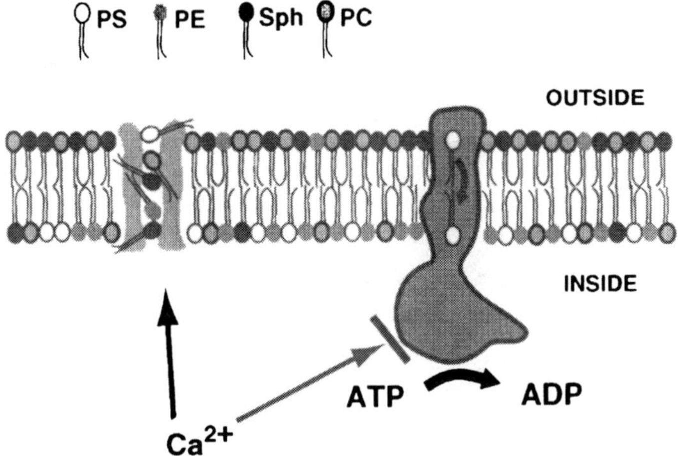

Fig. 6.1. Proteins that regulate transbilayer distribution of phospholipids. At left, the scramblase is activated by Ca^{2+}; at right, the ATP-dependent aminophospholipid translocase is inactivated by Ca^{2+}. Aminophospholipids include phosphatidylserine (PS) and phosphatidylethanolamine (PE); choline phospholipids include phosphatidylcholine (PC) and sphingomyelin (Sph).

cells. After a 10 min incubation to allow transport, dithionite was added to a concentration that reduced all external probe within 30 s, and fluorescence was recorded continuously. The difference in fluorescence at 30 s between cells labeled with an analog of PS and cells labeled with an analog of the zwitterion phosphatidylcholine (PC) represents PS internalized by the translocase and thereby inaccessible to reduc-

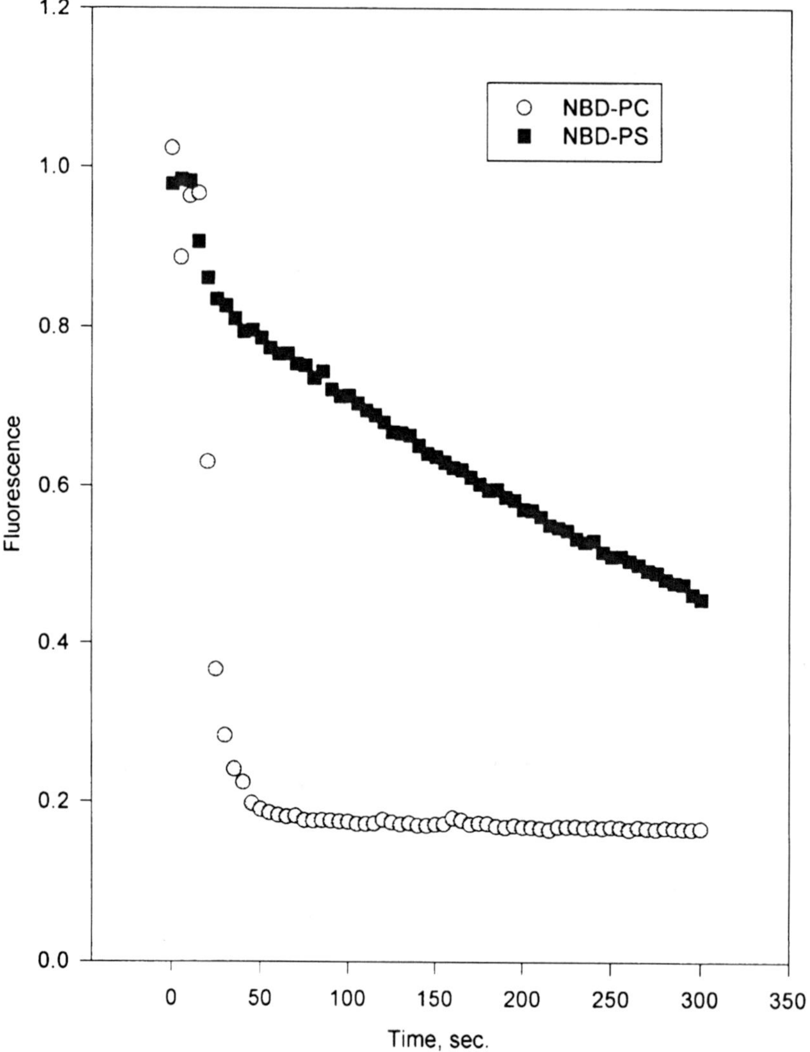

Fig. 6.2. Measuring translocase activity. DO11.10 *T* lymphocyte hybridoma cells were incubated at 37°C for 10 min in the presence of PS or PC labeled with 7-nitro-2,1,3-benzoxadiazol-4-yl (NBD). The cells were then transferred to a fluorimeter, 2 mM sodium dithionite added, and fluorescence recorded continuously.

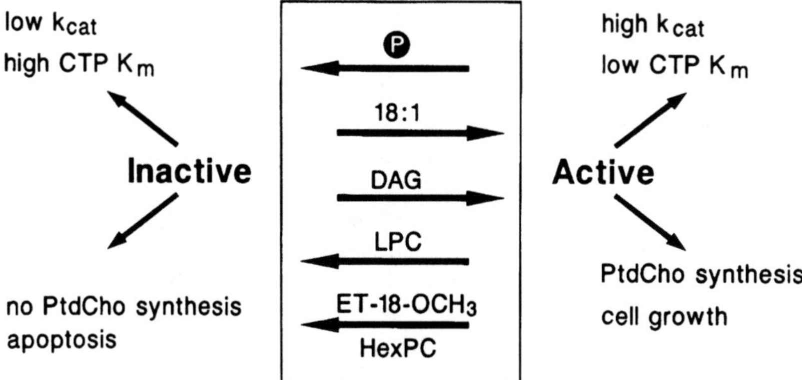

Fig. 4.8. Regulation of CT by physiological signals and antineoplastic phospholipids. Positive activators of CT are lipids such as oleic acid (18:1) and diacylglycerol (DAG). CT is negatively regulated by phosphorylation and lipid modulators LPC and ET-18-OCH$_3$. Inactivation of CT is due to a decrease in the affinity of the enzyme for CTP and results in decreased PtdCho synthesis followed by apoptosis. CT activation is associated with a higher affinity for CTP and increase in PtdCho synthesis and cell growth.

LPC restores PtdCho synthesis and prevents apoptosis in cells treated with ET-18-OCH$_3$ (69), we proposed that the inhibition at CT triggers apoptosis and is the primary cause for the cytotoxicity of antineoplastic phospholipids. This view is reinforced by the recent demonstration that a CHO cell line with a temperature-sensitive mutation in CT undergoes apoptosis at the nonpermissive temperature (77), thus confirming that blockage of PtdCho synthesis at CT can account for the cytotoxic effect of ET-18-OCH$_3$. Although exogenous LPC restores viability to cells, ET-18-OCH$_3$ still causes growth stasis when apoptosis is prevented (69), indicating that there is a second site for ET-18-OCH$_3$ action that results in cell cycle arrest. Major issues that will be addressed are whether the other members of the antineoplastic phospholipid class also target CT as the major component of their cytotoxic action and the identification of the second target for ET-18-OCH$_3$ that is responsible for growth arrest.

Acknowledgments

This work was supported by National Institutes of Health grant GM 45737 (to S. J.), Cancer Center (CORE) support grant CA 21765, and the American Lebanese Syrian Associated Charities.

References

1. Kudo, I., Nojima, S., Chang, H.W., Yanoshita, R., Hayashi, H., Kondo, E., Nomura, H., and Inoue, K. (1987) Antitumor Activity of Synthetic Alkylphospholipids with or without PAF Activity, *Lipids 22*, 862–867.

2. Westphal, O. (1987) Ether lipids in Oncology—Welcoming Address, *Lipids 22*, 787–788.

3. Munder, P.G., Weltzein, H.U., and Modolell, M. (1977) Lysolecithin and the Action of Complement, *Immunol. 7*, 411–424.

4. Berdel, W.E., Bausert, W.R.E., Weltzein, H.U., Modolell, M.L., Sidman, K.H., and Munder, P.G. (1980) The Influence of Alkyl-Lysophospholipids and Lysophospholipid-Activated Macrophages on the Development of Metastasis of 3-Lewis Lung Carcinoma, *Eur. J. Cancer 16*, 1119–1204.

5. Runge, M.H., Andreesen, R., Pfleidrer. A., and Munder, P.G. (1980) Destruction of Human Solid Tumors by Alkyl Lysophospholipids, *J. Natl. Cancer Inst. 64*, 1301–1306.

6. Andreesen, R., Modolell, M., Weltzein. H.U., Eibl, H., Common, H.H., Lohr, G.W., and Munder, P.G. (1978) Selective Destruction of Human Leukemic Cells by Alkyl-Lysophospholipids, *Cancer Res. 38*, 3894–3899.

7. Hoffman, D.R., Hoffman, L.H., and Snyder. F. (1986) Cytotoxicity and Metabolism of Alkyl Phospholipid Analogues in Neoplastic Cells, *Cancer Res. 46*, 5803–5809.

8. Vallari, D.S., Record, M., Smith. Z.L., and Snyder, F. (1989) *O*-alkyl-*O*-methylglyc-erophosphocholine, an Antineoplastic Lipid. Undergoes Spontaneous Redistribution between Biological Membranes Prepared from HL-60 Cells, *Biochim. Biophys. Acta 1006*, 250–254.

9. Vogler, W.R., Olson, A.C., Okamoto. S., Shoji, M., Raynoe, R.L., Kuo, J.F., Berdel, W.E., Eibl, H., Hajdu, J., and Nomura. H. (1991) Comparison of Selective Cytotoxicity of Alkyl Lysophospholipids, *Lipids 26*, 1418–1423.

10. Noseda, A., Berens, M.E., Piantadosi. C., and Modest, E.J. (1987) Neoplastic Cell Inhibition with New Ether Lipid Analogs, *Lipids 22*, 878–883.

11. Andreesen, R., Modolell, M., and Munder. P.G. (1979) Selective Sensitivity of Chronic Myelogenous Leukemia Cell Populations to Alkyl-Lysophospholipids, *Blood 54*, 519–523.

12. Berdel, W.E. (1991) Membrane-Interactive Lipids as Experimental Anticancer Drugs, *Br. J. Cancer 64*, 208–211.

13. Vogler, W.R., and Berdel, W.E. (1993) Autologous Bone Marrow Transplantation with Alkyl-Lysophospholipid-Purged Marrow, *J. Hematother. 2*, 93–102.

14. Vogler, W.R. (1994) Bone Marrow Purging in Acute Leukemia with Alkyl-Lysophospholipids: A New Family of Anticancer Drugs, *Leuk. Lymphoma 13*, 53–60.

15. Daniel, L.W. (1993) in *Cancer Chemotherapy*, Hickman, J.A., and Tritton, T.R., eds., Blackwell Scientific, Oxford, pp. 146–178.

16. Noseda, A., White, J.G., Godwin. P.L., Jerome, W.G., and Modest, E.J. (1989) Effect of Anti-Neoplastic Ether Lipids on Model and Biological Membranes, *Exp. Molec. Pathol. 50*, 69–83.

17. Vallari, D.S., Austinhirst, R., and Snyder. F. (1990) Development of Specific Functionally Active Receptors for Platelet-Activating Factor in HL-60 Cells Following Granulocytic Differentiation, *J. Biol. Chem. 265*, 4261–4265.

18. Workman, P., Donaldson, J., and Lohmeyer, M. (1990) Platelet-Activating Factor (PAF) Antagonist WEB 2086 Does Not Modulate the Cytotoxicity of PAF or Antitumor Alkyl Lysophospholipids ET-18-O-Methyl and SRI 62-834 in HL-60 Promyelocytic Leukaemia Cells, *Biochem. Pharmacol. 41*, 319–322.

19. Salari, H., Dryden, P., Howard. S., and Bittman, R. (1992) Two Different Sites of Action for Platelet Activating Factor and 1-*O*-alkyl-2-*O*-methyl-*sn*-glycero-3-phosphocholine on Platelets and Leukemic Cells, *Biochem. Cell Biol. 70*, 129–135.

20. Parker, J., Daniel, L.W., and Waite, M. (1987) Evidence of Protein Kinase C Involvement in Phorbol Diester-Stimulated Arachidonic Acid Release and Prostaglandin Synthesis, *J. Biol. Chem. 262*, 5358–5393.
21. Heesbeen E.C., Verdonck, L.F., Haagmans, M., van Heugten, H.G., Staal, G.E.J., and Ruksen, G. (1993) Adsorption and Uptake of the Alkyllysophospholipid ET-18-OCH₃ by HL-60 Cells during Induction of Differentiation by Dimethylsulfoxide, *Leuk. Res. 17*, 143–148.
22. Salari, H., Dryden, P., Davenport, R., Howard, S., Kones, K., and Bittman, R. (1992) Inhibition of Protein Kinase C by Ether-Linked Lipids Is Not Correlated with Their Antineoplastic Activity on WEHI-3B and R6X-B15 Cells, *Biochim. Biophys. Acta 1134*, 81–88.
23. Heesbeen, E.C., Verdonck, L.F., Staal, G.E., and Rijksen, G. (1994) Protein Kinase C Is Not Involved in the Cytotoxic Action of 1-octadecyl-2-*O*-methyl-*sn*-glycerol-3-phosphocholine in HL-60 and K562 Cells, *Biochem. Pharmacol. 47*, 1481–1488.
24. Powis, G., Seewald, M.J., Gratas, C., Melder, D., Riebow, J., and Modest, E.J. (1992) Selective Inhibition of Phosphatidylinositol Phospholipase C by Cytotoxic Ether Lipid Analogues, *Cancer Res. 52*, 2835–2840.
25. Seewald, M.J., Olsen, R.A., Sehgal, I., Melder, D.C., Modest, E.J., and Powis, G. (1990) Inhibition of Growth Factor-Dependent Inositol Phosphate Ca^{2+} Signaling by Antitumor Ether Lipid Analogues, *Cancer Res. 50*, 4458–4463.
26. Rabinowitch, H.D., Sklan, D., Chace, D.H., Stevens, R.D., and Fridovich, I. (1993) *Escherichia coli* Produces Linoleic Acid during Late Stationary Phase, *J. Bacteriol. 175*, 5324–5328.
27. Vance, D.E. (1989) in *Phosphatidylcholine Metabolism*, Vance, D.E., ed., CRC Press, Boca Raton, Florida, pp. 225–239.
28. Kent, C. (1990) Regulation of Phosphatidylcholine Biosynthesis, *Prog. Lipid Res. 29*, 87–105.
29. Kent, C. (1995) Eukaryotic Phospholipid Biosynthesis, *Annu. Rev. Biochem. 64*, 315–343.
30. Esko, J.D., Wermuth, M.M., and Raetz, C.R.H. (1981) Thermolabile CDP-Choline Synthetase in an Animal Cell Mutant Defective in Lecithin Formation, *J. Biol. Chem. 256*, 7388–7393.
31. Voelker, D.R. and Kennedy, E.P. (1982) Cellular and Enzymic Synthesis of Sphingomyelin, *Biochemistry 21*, 2753–2759.
32. Voelker, D.R. (1984) Phosphatidylserine Functions as the Major Precursor of Phosphatidylethanolamine in Cultured BHK 21 Cells, *Proc. Natl. Acad. Sci. USA 81*, 2669–2673.
33. Cornell, R., and Vance, D.E. (1987) Binding of CTP:Phosphocholine Cytidylyltransferase to Large Unilamellar Vesicles, *Biochim. Biophys. Acta 919*, 37–48.
34. Cornell, R.B. (1991) Regulation of CTP:Phospocholine Cytidylyltransferase by Lipids. 1. Negative Surface Charge Dependence for Activation, *Biochemistry 30*, 5873–5880.
35. Cornell, R.B. (1991) Regulation of CTP:Phosphocholine Cytidylyltransferase by Lipids. 2. Surface Curvature, Acyl Chain Length, and Lipid-Phase Dependence for Activation, *Biochemistry 30*, 5881–5888.
36. Sleight, R., and Kent, C. (1983) Regulation of Phosphatidylcholine Biosynthesis in Mammalian Cells. II. Effects of Phospholipase C Treatment on the Activity and Subcellular Distribution of CTP:Phosphocholine Cytidylyltransferase in Chinese Hamster Ovary and LM cell lines, *J. Biol. Chem. 258*, 831–835.

37. Sleight, R., and Kent, C. (1983) Regulation of Phosphatidylcholine Biosynthesis in Mammalian Cells. III. Effects of Alterations in the Phospholipid Compositions of Chinese Hamster Ovary and LM Cells on the Activity and Distribution of CTP:Phosphocholine Cytidylyltransferase, *J. Biol. Chem. 258*, 836–839.

38. Wright, P.S., Morand, J.N., and Kent, C. (1985) Regulation of Phosphatidylcholine Biosynthesis in Chinese Hamster Ovary Cells by Reversible Membrane Association of CTP:Phosphocholine Cytidylyltransferase, *J. Biol. Chem. 260*, 7919–7926.

39. Pelech, S.L., Cook, H.W., Paddon, H.B., and Vance, D.E. (1984) Membrane-Bound CTP:Phosphocholine Cytidylyltransferase Regulates the Rate of Phosphatidylcholine Synthesis in HeLa Cells Treated with Unsaturated Fatty Acids, *Biochim. Biophys. Acta 795*, 433–440.

40. Pelech, S.L., Pritchard, P.H., Brindley, D.N., and Vance, D.E. (1983) Fatty Acids Promote Translocation of CTP:Phosphocholine Cytidylyltransferase to the Endoplasmic Reticulum and Stimulate Rat Hepatic Phosphatidylcholine Synthesis, *J. Biol. Chem. 258*, 6782–6788.

41. Jamil, H., Yao, Z.M., and Vance, D.E. (1990) Feedback Regulation of CTP:Phosphocholine Cytidylyltransferase Translocation between Cytosol and Endoplasmic Reticulum by Phosphatidylcholine, *J. Biol. Chem. 265*, 4332–4339.

42. Jamil, H., and Vance, D.E. (1990) Head-Group Specificity for Feedback Regulation of CTP:Phosphocholine Cytidylyltransferase, *Biochem. J. 270*, 749–754.

43. Yao, Z.M., Jamil, H., and Vance, D.E. (1990) Choline Deficiency Causes Translocation of CTP:Phosphocholine Cytidylyltransferase from Cytosol to Endoplasmic Reticulum in Rat Liver, *J. Biol. Chem. 265*, 4326–4331.

44. Jamil, H., Hatch, G.M., and Vance, D.E. (1993) Evidence That Binding of CTP:Phosphocholine Cytidylyltransferase to Membranes in Rat Hepatocytes Is Modulated by the Ratio of Bilayer- to Non-Bilayer-Forming Lipids, *Biochem. J. 291*, 419–427.

45. Yang, W., Boggs, K.P., and Jackowski, S. (1996) The Association of Lipid Activators with the Amphipathic Helical Domain of CTP:Phosphocholine Cytidylyltransferase Accelerates Catalysis by Increasing the Affinity of the Enzyme for CTP, *J. Biol. Chem. 270*, 23951–23957.

46. Kalmar, G.B., Kay, R.J., Lachance, A., Aebersold, R., and Cornell, R.B. (1990) Cloning and Expression of Rat Liver CTP:Phosphocholine Cytidylyltransferase: An Amphipathic Protein That Controls Phosphatidylcholine Synthesis, *Proc. Natl. Acad. Sci. USA 87*, 6029–6033.

47. Craig, L., Johnson, J.E., and Cornell, R.B. (1994) Identification of the Membrane-Binding Domain of Rat Liver CTP:Phosphocholine Cytidylyltransferase Using Chymotrypsin Proteolysis, *J. Biol. Chem. 269*, 3311–3317.

48. Wang, Y., and Kent, C. (1995) Identification of an Inhibitory Domain of CTP:Phosphocholine Cytidylyltransferase, *J. Biol. Chem. 270*, 18948–18952.

49. Wieder, T., Geilen, C.C., Wieprecht, M., Becker, A., and Orfanos, C.E. (1994) Identification of a Putative Membrane-Interacting Domain of CTP:Phosphocholine Cytidylyltransferase from Rat Liver, *FEBS Lett. 345*, 207–210.

50. MacDonald, J.I.S., and Kent, C. (1994) Identification of Phosphorylation Sites in Rat Liver CTP:Phosphocholine Cytidylyltransferase, *J. Biol. Chem. 269*, 10529–10537.

51. Yang, W., and Jackowski, S. (1995) Lipid Activation of CTP:Phosphocholine Cytidylyltransferase Is Regulated by the Phosphorylated Carboxy Terminal Domain, *J. Biol. Chem. 270*, 16503–16506.

52. Watkins, J.D. and Kent, C. (1991) Regulation of CTP:Phosphocholine Cytidylyltransferase Activity and Subcellular Location by Phosphorylation in Chinese Hamster Ovary Cells, *J. Biol. Chem. 266*, 21113–21117.

53. Wang, Y., MacDonald, J.I.S., and Kent, C. (1993) Regulation of CTP:Phosphocholine Cytidylyltransferase in HeLa Cells, *J. Biol. Chem. 268*, 5512–5518.

54. Hatch, G.M., Jamil, H., Utal, A.K., and Vance, D.E. (1992) On the Mechanism of the Okadaic Acid-Induced Inhibition of Phosphatidylcholine Biosynthesis in Isolated Rat Hepatocytes, *J. Biol. Chem. 267*, 15751–15758.

55. Watkins, J.D., Wang, Y., and Kent, C. (1992) Regulation of CTP:Phosphocholine Cytidylyltransferase Activity and Phosphorylation in Rat Hepatocytes: Lack of Effect of Elevated cAMP Levels, *Arch. Biochem. Biophys. 292*, 360–367.

56. Sweitzer, T.D., and Kent, C. (1994) Expression of Wild-Type and Mutant Rat Liver CTP:Phosphocholine Cytidylyltransferase in a Cytidylyltransferase-Deficient Chinese Hamster Ovary Cell Line, *Arch. Biochem. Biophys. 311*, 107–116.

57. Houweling, M., Jamil, H., Hatch, G.M., and Vance, D.E. (1994) Dephosphorylation of CTP:Phosphocholine Cytidylyltransferase Is Not Required for Binding to Membranes, *J. Biol. Chem. 269*, 7544–7551.

58. Boggs, K.P., Rock, C.O., and Jackowski, S. (1995) Lysophosphatidylcholine and 1-*O*-octadecyl-2-*O*-methyl-*rac*-glycero-3-phosphocholine Inhibit the CDP-Choline Pathway of Phosphatidylcholine Synthesis at the CTP:Phosphocholine Cytidylyltransferase Step, *J. Biol. Chem. 270*, 7757–7764.

59. Besterman, J.M., and Domanico, P.L. (1992) Association and Metabolism of Exogenously-Derived Lysophosphatidylcholine by Cultured Mammalian Cells: Kinetics and Mechanisms, *Biochemistry 31*, 2046–2056.

60. Modolell, M., Andreesen, R., Pahlke, W., Brugger, U., and Munder, P.G. (1979) Disturbance of Phospholipid Metabolism during the Selective Destruction of Tumor Cells Induced by Alkyl-Lysophospholipids, *Cancer Res. 39*, 4681–4686.

61. Vogler, W.R., Whigham, E., Bennett, W.D., and Olson, A.C. (1985) Effect of Alkyl-Lysophospholipids on Phosphatidylcholine Biosynthesis in Leukemic Cell Lines, *Exp. Hematol. 13*, 629–633.

62. Herrmann, D.B.J. (1985) Changes in Cellular Lipid Synthesis of Normal and Neoplastic Cells during Cytolysis Induced by Alkyl Lysophospholipid Analogues, *J. Natl. Cancer Inst. 75*, 423–430.

63. Hoffman, D.R., Thomas, V.L., and Snyder, F. (1992) Inhibition of Cellular Transport Systems by Alkyl Phospholipid Analogs in HL-60 Human Leukemia Cells, *Biochim. Biophys. Acta 1127*, 74–80.

64. Tronchère, H., Tercé, F., Record, M., Ribbes, G., and Chap, H. (1991) Modulation of CTP:Phosphocholine Cytidylyltransferase Translocation by Oleic Acid and the Antitumoral Alkylphospholipid in HL-60 Cells, *Biochem. Biophys. Res. Commun. 176*, 157–165.

65. Geilen, C.C., Wieder, T., and Reutter, W. (1992) Hexadecylphosphocholine Inhibits Translocation of CTP:Choline-Phosphate Cytidylyltransferase in Madin-Darby Canine Kidney Cells, *J. Biol. Chem. 267*, 6719–6724.

66. Geilen, C.C., Wieder, T., Haase, A., Reutter, W., Morré, D.M., and Morré, D.J. (1994) Uptake, Subcellular Distribution and Metabolism of the Phospholipid Analogue Hexadecylphosphocholine in MDCK Cells, *Biochim. Biophys. Acta 1211*, 14–22.

67. Wieder, T., Geilen, C.C., and Reutter, W. (1993) Antagonism of Phorbol-Ester-Stimu-

lated Phosphatidylcholine Biosynthesis by the Phospholipid Analogue Hexadecylphosphocholine, *Biochem. J. 291*, 561–567.

68. Haase, R., Wieder, T., Geilen, C.C.. and Reutter, W. (1991) The Phospholipid Analogue Hexadecylphosphocholine Inhibits Phosphatidylcholine Biosynthesis in Madin-Darby Canine Kidney Cells, *FEBS. Lett. 288.* 129–132.

69. Boggs, K.P., Rock, C.O., and Jackowski. S. (1995) Lysophosphatidylcholine Attenuates the Cytotoxic Effects of the Antineoplastic Phospholipid 1-*O*-octadecyl-2-*O*-methyl-*rac*-glycero-3-phosphocholine. *J. Biol. Chem. 270,* 11612–11618.

70. Sohal, P.S., and Cornell, R.B. (1990) Sphingosine Inhibits the Activity of Rat Liver CTP:Phosphocholine Cytidylyltransferase. *J. Biol. Chem. 265,* 11746–11750.

71. Mollinedo, F., Martinez-Dalmau, R., and Modolell, M. (1993) Early and Selective Induction of Apoptosis in Human Leukemic Cells by the Alkyl-Lysophospholipid ET-18-OCH$_3$, *Biochem. Biophys. Res. Commun. 192*, 603–609.

72. Diomede, L., Colotta, F., Piovani, B., Re, F., Modest, E.J., and Samona, M. (1993) Induction of Apoptosis in Human Leukemic Cells by the Ether Lipid 1-Octadecyl-2-methyl-*rac*-glycero-3-phosphocholine. A Possible Basis for Its Selective Action, *Int. J. Cancer 53,* 124–130.

73. Surette, M.E., Winkler, J.D., Fonteh, A.N., and Chilton, F.H. (1996) Relationship Between Arachidonate-Phospholipid Remodeling and Apoptosis, *Biochemistry 35,* 9187–9196.

74. Esko, J.D., Nishijima, M., and Raetz, C.R.H. (1982) Animal Cells Dependent on Exogenous Phosphatidylcholine for Membrane Biogenesis, *Proc. Natl. Acad. Sci. USA 79,* 1698–1702.

75. Sugai, M., Chen, C.H., and Wu, H.C. (1992) Bacterial ADP-Ribosyltransferase with a Substrate Specificity of the Rho Protein Disassembles the Golgi Apparatus in Vero Cells and Mimics the Action of Brefeldin A, *Proc. Natl. Acad. Sci. USA 89,* 8903–8907.

76. Braun V. (1975) Covalent Lipoprotein from the Outer Membrane of *Escherichia coli, Biochim. Biophys. Acta 415,* 335–377.

77. Cui, Z., Houweling, M., Chen, M.H., Record, M., Chap, H., Vance, D.E., and Tercé, F. (1996) A Genetic Defect in Phosphatidylcholine Biosynthesis Triggers Apoptosis in Chinese Hamster Ovary Cells, *J. Biol. Chem. 271,* 14668–14671.

Chapter 5

Phosphoinositides, Phospholipase D, and Membrane Trafficking

Mordechai Liscovitch

Department of Biological Regulation, Weizmann Institute of Science, Rehovot 76100, Israel

Introduction

Lipid and lipid-derived messengers have in recent years been seen to form a previously unrecognized class of bioregulatory molecules, including 1,2-*sn*-diacylglycerol, inositol-1,4,5-trisphosphate, phosphatidylinositol-3,4,5-trisphosphate, phosphatidic acid, arachidonic acid, lysophosphatidylcholine, ceramide, and sphingosine-1-phosphate (1–3). These messenger molecules are produced by phospholipases and lipid kinases whose activity is strictly regulated by extracellular signals acting *via* their cell-surface receptors. Our work has focused on one of of these signal-activated enzymes: phospholipase D (PLD). Several excellent reviews have recently provided nearly comprehensive coverage of the many questions touched upon by research in the PLD field (4–7), and detailed reviews of specific topics can be found in a special issue of *Chemistry and Physics of Lipids*, devoted in its entirety to PLD (8). The present chapter will concentrate on recent advances in our understanding of the regulation and function of PLD, with particular emphasis on its possible role(s) in signal transduction and membrane traffic.

Biochemical Properties of Eukaryotic Phospholipases D

PLD is a phosphodiesterase that cleaves the distal phosphodiester bond of phospholipids (e.g., phosphatidylcholine) to produce a water-soluble product, such as choline, and a simple phospholipid called phosphatidic acid (PA) (Fig. 5.1, right). The reaction catalyzed by PLD is considered to be a phosphatidyl transfer reaction in which the phospholipid substrate donates the phosphatidyl group to an alcoholic acceptor. Normally, PLD catalyzes a simple hydrolytic reaction, in which water acts as the phosphatidyl group acceptor. However, most PLDs are also capable of utilizing primary short-chain alcohols as phosphatidyl group acceptors (Fig. 5.1, left). The resultant lipid product in that case is the corresponding phosphatidic acid alkyl ester, or phosphatidylalcohol (9). The ability to produce phosphatidylalcohols is a very useful property of PLD, because of the exclusive production of these abnormal phospholipids by PLD. Furthermore, phosphatidylalcohols are relatively stable metabolically, and their basal level in cells or tissues is extremely low. In contrast, PLD's natural lipid product, PA, can also be produced *via* the *de novo* pathway of

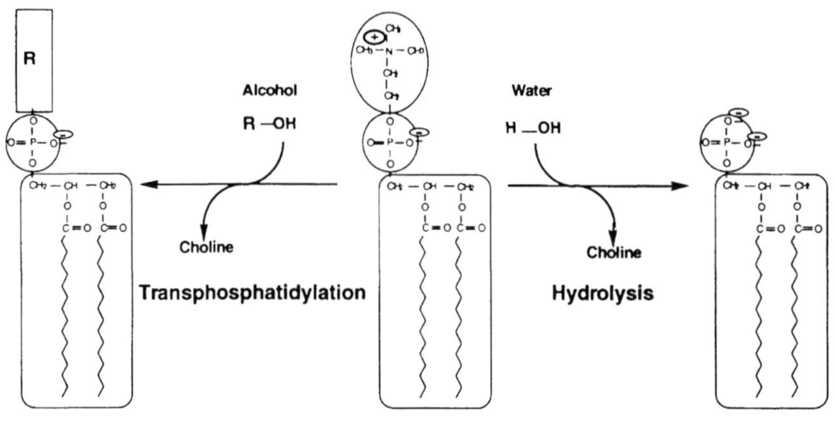

Fig. 5.1. Hydrolysis and transphosphatidylation reactions catalyzed by phospholipase D. PLD-type enzymes hydrolyze phospholipids such as phosphatidylcholine, resulting in the formation of phosphatidic acid and a free polar headgroup such as choline. Most PLDs also catalyze a transphosphatidylation reaction in which an an alcohol (R-OH, a short-chain primary alcohol such as methanol, ethanol, 1-propanol, or 1-butanol) serves as a phosphatidyl group acceptor, resulting in the production of a phosphatidyl-alcohol at the expense of PA.

phospholipid biosynthesis (i.e., by sequential acylation of glycerophosphate) and by a diacylglycerol kinase–mediated phosphorylation of diacylglycerol (DAG). Furthermore, PA can be quickly metabolized or utilized for subsequent synthesis of phosphatidylinositol and phosphatidylglycerol. Consequently, the formation of phosphatidylalcohols has been widely used as a specific marker for activation of PLD and was employed in a great many studies on the signal-activated nature of this enzyme.

The existence of multiple PLD isozymes in mammalian cells is suggested by a large body of data demonstrating the biochemical heterogeneity of different PLD preparations obtained from different organisms and tissues:

- A membrane-bound PLD activity, first identified in rat brain (10,11), was recently purified from pig lung and found to be a 190-kDa protein (12). This enzyme seems to be an integral membrane protein, is highly specific for phosphatidylcholine as substrate, and is activated by sodium oleate.

- A cytosolic PLD has also been identified and characterized (13–15). The cytosolic PLD is more permissive in its substrate interaction; it hydrolyzes phosphatidylethanolamine and phosphatidylinositol as well as phosphatidylcholine (13–15).

- An additional, membrane-bound PLD that behaves as a peripheral membrane protein was first described in HL-60 cell membranes (16) but is found also in porcine brain membranes (17). The peripheral membrane PLD is activated by the small guanine nucleotide–binding (G) protein ADP-ribosylation factor (ARF) (16,18). Indeed, two peaks of PLD activity were resolved by heparin–agarose chromatography of rat brain membrane extracts, corresponding to the oleate-dependent form and the ARF-dependent form (19). The ARF-dependent PLD can be found in Golgi-enriched membranes (20).

The existence of multiple PLD isozymes is likely related to the existence of diverse mechanisms of PLD activation and multiple functions of this enzyme. Recent evidence suggest that at least two small G proteins of the Ras superfamily can stimulate PLD activity. One of them is ARF (16,18,19), the other is RhoA (21,22), and they appear to interact with a cytosolic PLD and a membrane PLD, respectively (23). Another small G protein, Ral, may be coprecipitated with PLD, indicating that it is physically associated with the enzyme or with a tightly PLD-bound protein (24). Peripheral membrane and cytosolic forms of PLD may be related, because both may be activated by ARF. The exact nature of this relationship, if any, remains to be determined.

Putative Roles of Phospholipase D in Signal Transduction

The evidence showing that PLD is rapidly and dramatically activated in response to a wide variety of stimuli in many different cell types is overwhelming (4,6). The nature of the activating signals is diverse. Among the stimuli that activate PLD are hormones, growth factors, neurotransmitters, cytokines, extracellular matrix constituents, antigens, and certain physical stimuli such as radiation and mechanical stretch. In addition, PLD activity is stimulated by phorbol esters in virtually all cell types studied. These agents are activators of protein kinase C (PKC) isozymes. Hence, the activation of PKC is likely to be an upstream event in PLD activation. However, current evidence strongly supports the existence of PKC-independent pathway(s) of PLD activation in some cell types and the coexistence of PKC-dependent and PKC-independent activation of PLD by different agonists in the same cell type (e.g., Ref. 25). *In vitro* data on the interaction of PLD with different small GTPases and PKC isozymes support this conclusion.

Regardless of the mechanism of receptor–PLD coupling, the stimulation of PLD activity may be expected to have a number of immediate cellular consequences (Fig. 5.2).

- In cholinergic neurons, the action of a constitutively active phospholipase D–type activity was shown to provide choline, which was metabolically channeled to synthesis of the neurotransmitter acetylcholine (26).

- Phosphatidic acid produced by PLD may be converted into lysophosphatidic acid (LPA), a mitogenic factor present in serum (see Ref. 27 for review).

- Alternatively, PA may be dephosphorylated by phosphatidic acid phosphohydrolase (PAP) to form DAG. The possibility that PLD and PAP cooperate in providing the late-phase DAG for sustained activation of PKC has been reviewed (6).

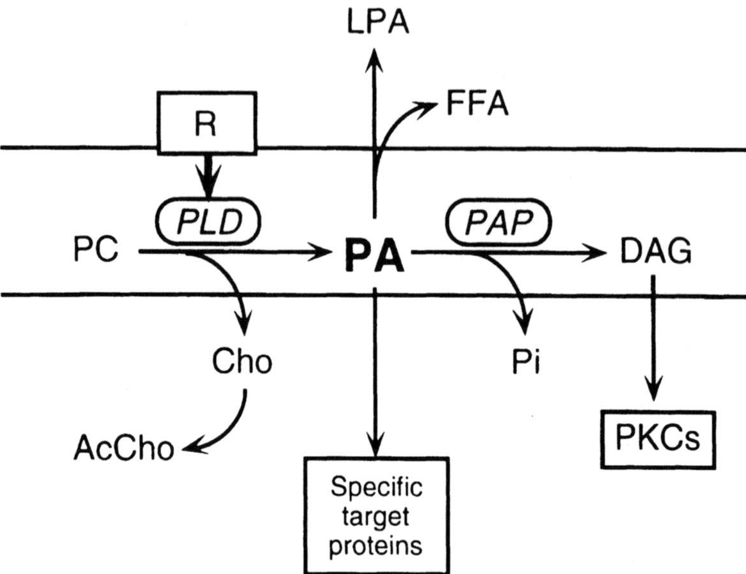

Fig. 5.2. The metabolism and putative signaling roles of phospholipase D products. Abbreviations: AcCho, acetylcholine; Cho, choline; DAG, diacylglycerol; FFA, free fatty acids; LPA, lysophosphatidic acid; PA, phosphatidic acid; PAP, phosphatidic acid phosphohydrolase; PC, phosphatidylcholine; Pi, inorganic phosphate; PKCs, protein kinase C isozymes; PLD, phospholipase D; R, cell surface receptor.

Finally, the evidence, albeit equivocal, that phosphatidic acid may itself act as an intracellular messenger is mounting rapidly. The activation of PLD results, under physiological conditions, in formation of PA (e.g., Ref. 28). In certain model systems (e.g., the human neutrophil), PA seems to satisfy all of Sutherland's classical criteria for a second messenger (29). However, physiological target proteins that are regulated by PA have not been identified with certainty. The activity of numerous enzymes and proteins is modulated by PA *in vitro*. These proteins are potential PA targets and include neutrophil NADPH oxidase (30), Ras GTPase activating protein (GAP) (31), an unidentified Ser/Thr kinase activity (32), certain protein kinase C isozymes (33,34), SH-protein tyrosine phosphatase 1 (35), *n*-chimaerin's *rac*-GAP activity (36), phospholipase C-γ (37), phosphatidylinositol-4-phosphate 5-kinase (38), and ADP-ribosylation factor (ARF) GAP (39). A recent study has shown that Raf-1, the upstream Ser/Thr kinase of the MAP kinase cascade, may be recruited to the membrane by binding to PA (40). However, to date none of these enzymes has been shown to be a *bona fide* target of PA *in situ*. Thus, the search for physiological PA targets continues.

Phosphatidylinositol-4,5-bisphosphate as a Cofactor of Phospholipase D

A neutral-active, oleate-dependent PLD was identified in rat brain membranes and characterized in our laboratory (11,41,42). This enzyme was partially purified and characterized kinetically (43). One of the striking properties of the rat brain PLD is its inhibition by aminoglycoside antibiotics, such as neomycin and its congeners (44). Because aminoglycosides have a very high affinity for acidic phospholipids (but none to positively charged phospholipids such as the PLD substrate PC), we proposed that negatively charged phospholipids act as essential cofactors of PLD (44). This hypothesis is supported by recent experiments with the highly acidic phospholipid phosphatidylinositol-4,5-bisphosphate (PIP_2) (45,46), which showed that PLD is greatly stimulated by PIP_2. The partially purified, oleate-dependent PLD is dramatically activated by low concentrations of PIP_2 when assayed in the absence of oleate, but not by other acidic phospholipids (45). Notably, the stimulatory effect of PIP_2 on the oleate-dependent PLD could not be observed when the PLD assay is carried out in the presence of sodium oleate (M. Liscovitch, unpublished results; cf. Ref. 19). Stimulation of PLD activity by PIP_2 required very low surface concentrations of PIP_2 (up to 5 mol%) and exhibited similar EC_{50} values (0.04–0.15 mol%), whether PLD activity was assayed in Triton X-100 micelles, pure C_6-NBD-PC micelles, or brain membrane particles (43). Thus, PIP_2 stimulates PLD activity at physiological concentrations that are normally found in biological membranes. Additional experiments have suggested that neomycin inhibits membrane PLD activity by interacting with endogenous PIP_2 (45). Taken together, these data suggest that PIP_2 may act as a cofactor of PLD.

The importance of PIP_2 in PLD activation was underscored by studies carried out in permeabilized U937 cells (46). One of the characteristics of PLD activation by guanosine 5'-3-O-(thio)triphosphate (GTPγS) in permeabilized cells is its marked potentiation by MgATP (e.g., Refs. 47,48). PIP_2 is synthesized by a sequential, ATP-dependent phosphorylation of phosphatidylinositol on the D-4 and D-5 positions of the inositol ring, catalyzed by phosphatidylinositol 4-kinase (PI4K) and phosphatidylinositol-4-phosphate 5-kinase (PIP5K), respectively. Our results raised the possibility that MgATP potentiates GTPγS-induced PLD activation by supporting production of PIP_2 in the cells, thus maintaining PIP_2 at a level sufficient for PLD activation. This hypothesis was tested in permeabilized U937 cells by using an inhibitory monoclonal antibody to PI4K (46). Initially, HPLC analysis of cellular PIP_2 levels confirmed that its formation is absolutely dependent on the presence of MgATP and that it is further increased by GTPγS. An inhibitory anti-PI4K (Ab 4C5G) inhibited phosphatidylinositol-4-phosphate and PIP_2 synthesis in the cells by 80% and completely abolished the activation of PLD, proving that PIP_2 synthesis is required for PLD activation (46). In a previous study (16) it had been reported that the ARF-dependent PLD is also stimulated by PIP_2 *in vitro*. Taken together, these studies suggest that both oleate-activated and ARF-activated PLDs are sensitive to

PIP$_2$ (Fig. 5.3). Recently we obtained evidence for the existence of at least two forms of PLD activity in yeast, one of which, Pld1, is sensitive to PIP$_2$ (49). In conclusion, current evidence suggests that the sensitivity to PIP$_2$ is a general property of most eukaryotic PC-specific PLDs.

The results described above indicate that a causal link exists between phosphoinositide kinases that synthesize PIP$_2$ and PLD activation; furthermore, they suggest the possibility that these enzymes may act in concert in mediating PLD-dependent cellular events. It is important to note that PIP$_2$ has multiple functions in cells. It is a precursor of three other second messengers: 1,2-*sn*-diacylglycerol, inositol-1,4,5-trisphosphate, and phosphatidylinositol-3,4,5-trisphosphate; it binds to several actin-binding proteins such as gelsolin and profilin; and it interacts with a number of proteins associated with membrane traffic events. Thus, phosphoinositide kinases may play a significant role in coordinating the multiple cellular functions that depend on PIP$_2$.

Putative Functions of Phosphoinositides and Phospholipase D in Membrane Traffic

Of particular interest is the hypothesis that phosphoinositide kinases and PLD interact in the complex machinery that is responsible for vesicular trafficking. PLD has been implicated in membrane transport, since it has been identified as an ARF target (16,18). More recent studies have demonstrated that PLD is present in Golgi

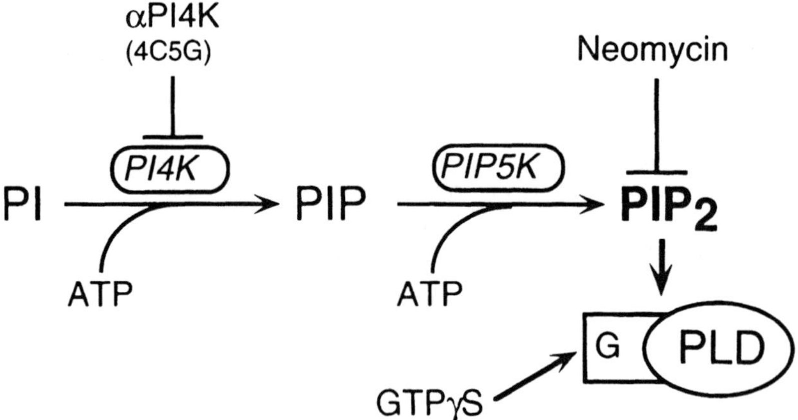

Fig. 5.3. Role of phosphatidylinositol-4,5-bisphosphate biosynthesis in PLD activation. Abbreviations: G, small GTPase; GTPγS, guanosine 5'-3-O-(thio)triphosphate; PI, phosphatidylinositol; PI4K, phosphatidylinositol 4-kinase; PIP, phosphatidylinositol-4-phosphate; PIP5K, phosphatidylinositol-4-phosphate 5-kinase; PIP$_2$, phosphatidylinositol-4,5-bisphosphate; PLD, phospholipase D.

membranes (20), and evidence was presented that PLD mediates ARF-dependent formation of coated vesicles (50). In addition, a remarkable convergence of evidence indicates that phosphoinositides, phosphoinositide kinases, and phosphatidylinositol transfer protein are linked to a variety of membrane traffic events (51,52). However, the exact details of such interaction, if it exists, as well as the mode of action of PA, the main lipid mediator produced by PLD, remain open for speculation (45,51). Phosphatidic acid could act by direct regulation of target proteins involved in vesicle targeting, docking, and fusion. In addition, under certain circumstances, the formation of phosphatidic acid may lead to changes in lipid bilayer properties that would facilitate vesicle budding and fusion events that occur in the course of intracellular membrane traffic. Future studies will likely prove or refute these exciting possibilities.

Identification and Disruption of Yeast *PLD1:* Properties of the PLD Gene Family

Purification of mammalian PC-specific PLD enzymes has proven to be a difficult task (but cf. Ref. 12), thus preventing cloning of PLD genes and delaying further understanding of their regulation and function. This impasse was overcome with the cloning of the first eukaryotic PC-PLD, from the plant *Ricinus communis* (53). The availability of PLD sequence information enabled sequence databanks to be screened for homologous sequences for the first time, resulting in identification of a yeast PLD gene (49,54,55) and a human ARF-dependent PLD gene (56). The yeast gene, *PLD1,* was originally sequenced in the course of the yeast genome project as an open reading frame denoted YKR031c, encoding a 195-kDa hypothetical protein of unknown function. Analyzing the Genbank database, using the BLAST algorithm with the sequence of plant PLD as probe, we discovered that YKR031c shared with plant PLD eight short but highly homologous segments that appeared in both sequences in the same order. We therefore postulated that YKR031c encodes a yeast PLD, tentatively named Pld1. Genetic disruption of *PLD1* was accomplished by replacing a central portion of the gene (which includes the most highly conserved region) with HIS3 as a selectable marker, followed by insertion of the disrupted gene into the yeast genome by homologous recombination. The disruption of *PLD1* resulted in a complete loss of PC-PLD activity in Pld1 lysates when the assay was carried out in the absence of calcium ions, demonstrating that *PLD1* encodes a calcium-independent PLD activity (49). Similar results were obtained in parallel studies by others (54,55). Recently we and others have found that yeast cells also express a calcium-dependent PLD activity whose properties are strikingly different from those of Pld1 (57,58).

Together, the plant, yeast, and human PLDs define a novel gene family. A schematic representation of the structure of those three members of the PLD family is shown in Fig. 5.4. It may be readily seen that the overall homology among these proteins is very low. However, some regions are conserved in all three sequences, whereas others are conserved only in the yeast and human PLDs. The plant PLD has

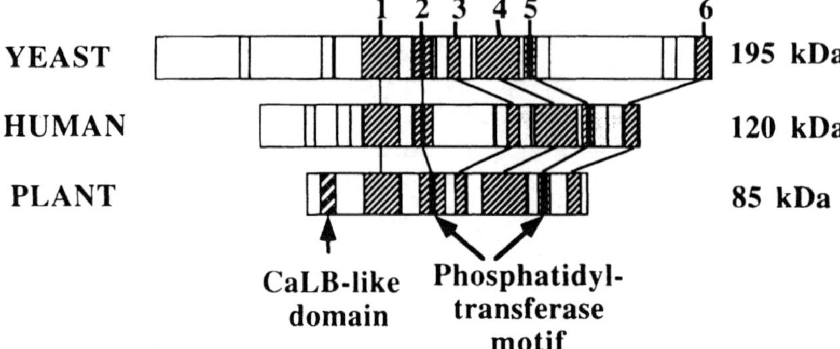

Fig. 5.4. Domain structure of eukaryotic PC-PLDs. Yeast, human, and plant PLD sequences were aligned according to multiple BLAST analyses with each of the sequences as query. Domains that are conserved in all three proteins are hatched; domains that are found in yeast and human PLDs are shaded. The phosphatidyltransferase motif, found in both prokaryotic and eukaryotic PLDs as well as in non–PLD phosphatidyltransferases, is shown in black. The Ca^{2+}-lipid binding (CaLB) domain, present only in plant PLD, is crosshatched.

a calcium-lipid binding domain that is not to be found in the other PLDs. All PLDs have a relatively short motif, termed the phosphatidyltransferase motif, which they share with certain phospholipid synthases that, like PLD, have a phosphatidyl transfer-based reaction mechanism. It may be speculated that the highly conserved domains are important for the catalytic activity of PLD, whereas the nonconserved regions represent regulatory domains that may participate in interactions with protein and lipid cofactors. Future structure–function analyses with recombinant mutated enzymes and enzyme fragments are likely to establish the specific functions associated with the different domains.

Conclusion

After more than a decade in which research on PLD was limited by the lack of molecular tools, the cloning and sequencing of the first eukaryotic PLDs opens a new era in which rapid progress in understanding the cellular and molecular biology of PLD may be expected. A number of major issues remain to be resolved, including the mechanisms of PLD activation and the identity of the cellular proteins targeted by PA. Identification of upstream regulators of PLD and downstream effectors is likely to help elucidate the function(s) of the different PLD isoforms in signal transduction and membrane traffic.

Acknowledgments

The work described in this review was supported in part by grants from the Israel Science Foundation administered by the Israel Academy of Science and Humanities, the Minerva

Foundation (Munich, Germany), and the Leo and Julia Forchheimer Center for Molecular Genetics at the Weizmann Institute of Science.

References

1. Liscovitch, M., and Cantley, L.C. (1994) Lipid Second Messengers, *Cell 77,* 329–334.
2. Exton, J.H. (1994) Messenger Molecules Derived from Membrane Lipids, *Curr. Opin. Cell Biol. 6,* 226–229.
3. Nishizuka, Y. (1995) Protein Kinase C and Lipid Signaling for Sustained Cellular Responses, *FASEB J. 9,* 484–496.
4. Billah, M.M. (1993) Phospholipase D and Cell Signaling, *Curr. Opin. Immunol. 5,* 114–123.
5. Exton, J.H. (1994) Phosphatidylcholine Breakdown and Signal Transduction, *Biochim. Biophys. Acta 1212,* 26–42.
6. Liscovitch, M., and Chalifa, V. (1994) in *Signal-Activated Phospholipases,* Liscovitch, M., ed., R.G. Landes, Austin, Texas, pp. 31–63.
7. Klein, J., Chalifa, V., Liscovitch, M., and Loffelholz, K. (1995) Role of Phospholipase D Activation in Nervous System Physiology and Pathophysiology, *J. Neurochem. 65,* 1445–1455.
8. Natarajan, V.E. (1996) Phospholipase D and Signal Transduction in Mammalian Cells, *Chem. Phys. Lipids 80,* 1–142.
9. Heller, M. (1978) in *Advances in Lipid Research,* Paoletty, R., and Kritchevsky, D., eds., Academic Press, New York, pp. 267–326.
10. Kanfer, J.N. (1980) The Base Exchange Enzymes and Phospholipase D of Mammalian Tissue, *Canad. J. Biochem. 58,* 1370–1380.
11. Chalifa, V., Möhn, H., and Liscovitch, M. (1990) A Neutral Phospholipase D Activity from Rat Brain Synaptic Plasma Membranes. Identification and Partial Characterization, *J. Biol. Chem. 265,* 17512–17519.
12. Okamura, S., and Yamashita, S. (1994) Purification and Characterization of Phosphatidylcholine Phospholipase D from Pig Lung, *J. Biol. Chem. 269,* 31207–31213.
13. Balsinde, J., Diez, E., Fernandez, B., and Mollinedo, F. (1989) Biochemical Characterization of Phospholipase D Activity from Human Neutrophils, *Europ. J. Biochem. 186,* 717–724.
14. Wang, P., Anthes, J.C., Siegel, I.M., Egan, R.W., and Billah, M.M. (1991) Existence of Cytosolic Phospholipase D. Identification and Comparison with Membrane-Bound Enzyme, *J. Biol. Chem. 266,* 14877–14880.
15. Huang, C., Wykle, R.L., Daniel, L., and Cabot, M.C. (1992). Identification of Phosphatidylcholine-Selective and Phosphatidylinositol-Selective Phospholipase D in Madin-Darby Canine Kidney Cells, *J. Biol. Chem. 267,* 16859–16865.
16. Brown, H.A., Gutowski, S., Moomaw, C.R., Slaughter, C., and Sternweis, P.C. (1993) ADP-Ribosylation Factor, a Small GTP-Dependent Regulatory Protein, Stimulates Phospholipase D Activity, *Cell 75,* 1137–1144.
17. Brown, H.A., Gutowski, S., Kahn, R.A., and Sternweis, P.C. (1995) Partial Purification and Characterization of ARF-Sensitive Phospholipase D from Porcine Brain, *J. Biol. Chem. 270,* 14935–14943.
18. Cockcroft, S. (1994) in *Signal-Activated Phospholipases,* Liscovitch, M., ed., R.G. Landes, Austin, Texas, pp. 65–83.

19. Massenburg, D., Han, J.-S., Liyanage, M., Patton, W.A., Rhee, S.G., Moss, J., and Vaughan, M. (1994) Activation of Rat Brain Phospholipase D by ADP-Ribosylation Factors 1, 5, and 6: Separation of ADP-Ribosylation Factor-Dependent and Oleate-Dependent Enzymes, *Proc. Natl. Acad. Sci. USA 91*, 11718–11722.

20. Ktistakis, N.T., Brown, H.A., Sternweis, P.C., and Roth, M.G. (1995) Phospholipase D Is Present in Golgi-Enriched Membranes and Its Activation by ADP-Ribosylation Factor is Sensitive to Brefeldin A, *Proc. Natl. Acad. Sci. USA 92*, 4952–4956.

21. Bowman, E.P., Uhlinger, D.J., and Lambeth, J.D. (1993) Neutrophil Phospholipase D Is Activated by a Membrane-Associated Rho Family Small Molecular Weight GTP-Binding Protein, *J. Biol. Chem. 268*, 21509–21512.

22. Malcolm, K.C., Ross, A.H., Qiu, R.-G., Symons, M., and Exton, J.H. (1994) Activation of Rat Liver Phospholipase D by the Small GTP-Binding Protein RhoA, *J. Biol. Chem. 269*, 25951–25954.

23. Siddiqui, A.R., Smith, J.L., Ross, A.H., Qiu, R.-G., Symons, M., and Exton, J.H. (1995) Regulation of Phospholipase D in HL60 Cells. Evidence for a Cytosolic Phospholipase D. *J. Biol. Chem. 270*, 8466–8473.

24. Jiang, H., Luo, J.-Q., Urano, T., Frankel, P., Lu, Z., Foster, D.A., and Feig, L.A. (1995) Involvement of Ral GTPase in v-Src-Induced Phospholipase D Activation, *Nature 378*, 409–412.

25. Ben-Av, P., Eli, Y., Schmidt, U.S., Tobias, K., and Liscovitch, M. (1993) Distinct Mechanisms of Phospholipase D Activation and Attenuation Utilized by Different Mitogens in NIH-3T3 Fibroblasts, *Europ. J. Biochem. 215*, 455–463.

26. Lee, H.C., Fellenz, M.P., Liscovitch, M., and Blusztajn, J.K. (1993) A Phospholipase D-Catalyzed Hydrolysis of Phosphatidylcholine Provides the Choline Precursor for Acetylcholine Synthesis in a Human Neuronal Cell Line, LA-N-2, *Proc. Natl. Acad. Sci. USA 90*, 10086–10090.

27. Moolenaar, W.H. (1995) Lysophosphatidic Acid, a Multifunctional Lipid Messenger, *J. Biol. Chem. 270*, 12949–12952.

28. Fukami, K., and Takenawa, T. (1992) Phosphatidic Acid That Accumulates in Platelet-Derived Growth Factor-Stimulated Balb/c 3T3 Cells Is a Potential Mitogenic Signal, *J. Biol. Chem. 267*, 10988–10993.

29. English, D., Cui, Y., and Siddiqui, R.A. (1996) Messenger Functions of Phosphatidic Acid, *Chem. Phys. Lipids 80*, 117–132.

30. Bellavite, P., Corso, F., Dusi, S., Grzeskowiak, M., Della-Bianca, V., and Rossi, F. (1988) Activation of NADPH-Dependent Superoxide Production in Plasma Membrane Extracts of Pig Neutrophils by Phosphatidic Acid, *J. Biol. Chem. 263*, 8210–8214.

31. Tsai, M.H., Yu, C.L., Wei, F.S., and Stacey, D.W. (1989) The Effect of GTPase Activating Protein upon Ras Is Inhibited by Mitogenically Responsive Lipids, *Science 243*, 522–526.

32. Bocckino, S.B., Wilson, P.B., and Exton, J.H. (1991). Phosphatidate-Dependent Protein Phosphorylation, *Proc. Natl. Acad. Sci. USA 88*, 5210–6213.

33. Ballas, L., Meyer, M., Burns, D., and Loomis, C. (1993) Lipid Activators of Protein Kinase C-η: Characterization of Specific Phosphatidic Acid Activators, *FASEB J. 7*, A1120.

34. Limatola, C., Schaap, D., Moolenaar, W.H., and van Blitterswijk, W. (1994) Phosphatidic Acid Activation of Protein Kinase C-ζ Overexpressed in COS Cells: Comparison with Other Protein Kinase C Isotypes and Other Acidic Lipids, *Biochem. J. 304*, 1001–1008.

35. Zhao, Z., Shen, S.-H., and Fischer, E.H. (1993) Stimulation by Phospholipids of a Protein-Tyrosine-Phosphatase Containing Two *src* Homology 2 Domains, *Proc. Natl. Acad. Sci. USA 90*, 4251–4255.

36. Ahmed, S., Lee, J., Kozma, R., Best, A., Monfries, C., and Lim, L. (1993) A Novel Functional Target for Tumor-Promoting Phorbol Esters and Lysophosphatidic Acid. The p21*rac*-GTPase Activating Protein *n*-Chimaerin, *J. Biol. Chem. 268*, 10709–10712.

37. Jones, G.A., and Carpenter, G. (1993) The Regulation of Phospholipase C-γ by Phosphatidic Acid. Assessment of Kinetic Parameters, *J. Biol. Chem. 268*, 20845–20850.

38. Jenkins, G.H., Fisette, P.L., and Anderson, R.A. (1994) Type I Phosphatidylinositol 4-Phosphate 5-Kinase Isoforms Are Specifically Stimulated by Phosphatidic Acid, *J. Biol. Chem. 269*, 11547–11554.

39. Randazzo, P.A., and Kahn, R.A. (1994) GTP Hydrolysis by ADP-Ribosylation Factor Is Dependent on Both an ADP-Ribosylation Factor GTPase-Activating Protein and Acid Phospholipids, *J. Biol. Chem. 269*, 10758–10763.

40. Ghosh, S., Strum, J.C., Sciorra, V.A., Daniel, L., and Bell, R.M. (1996). Raf-1 Kinase Possesses Distinct Binding Domains for Phosphatidylserine and Phosphatidic Acid. Phosphatidic Acid Regulates the Translocation of Raf-1 in 12-*O*-tetradecanoylphorbol-13-acetate-Stimulated Madin-Darby Canine Kidney Cells, *J. Biol. Chem. 271*, 8472–8480.

41. Möhn, H., Chalifa, V., and Liscovitch, M. (1992). Substrate Specificity of Neural Phospholipase D from Rat Brain Studied by Selective Labeling of Endogenous Synaptic Membrane Phospholipids *in vitro*, *J. Biol. Chem. 267*, 11131–11136.

42. Danin, M., Chalifa, V., Möhn, H., Schmidt, U.S., and Liscovitch, M. (1993) in *Lipid Metabolism in Signaling Systems*, Fain, J.N., ed., Academic Press, San Diego, California, pp. 14–24.

43. Chalifa-Caspi, V., Eli, Y., and Liscovitch, M. (1998) Kinetic Analysis of Partially Purified Rat Brain Phospholipase D Activity in Mixed Micelles. Activation by Phosphatidylinositol 4,5-Bisphosphate, *Neurochem. Res. 23*, 589–599.

44. Liscovitch, M., Chalifa, V., Danin, M., and Eli, Y. (1991) Inhibition of Neural Phospholipase D Activity by Aminoglycoside Antibiotics, *Biochem. J. 279*, 319–321.

45. Liscovitch, M., Chalifa, V., Pertile, P., Chen, C.-S., and Cantley, L.C. (1994) Novel Function of Phosphatidylinositol 4,5-Bisphosphate as a Cofactor for Brain Membrane Phospholipase D, *J. Biol. Chem. 269*, 21403–21406.

46. Pertile, P., Liscovitch, M., Chalifa, V., and Cantley, L.C. (1995) Phosphatidylinositol 4,5-Bisphosphate Synthesis Is Required for Activation of Phospholipase D in U937 Cells, *J. Biol. Chem. 270*, 5130–5135.

47. Liscovitch, M., and Eli, Y. (1991) Ca2+ Inhibits Guanine Nucleotide-Activated Phospholipase D in Neural-Derived NG108-15 Cells, *Cell Regul. 2*, 1011–1019.

48. Kanoh, H., Kanaho, Y., and Nozawa, Y. (1993) Requirement of Adenosine 5′-Triphosphate and Ca^{2+} for Guanosine 5′-Triphosphate-Binding Protein-Mediated Phospholipase D Activation in Rat Pheochromocytoma PC 12 Cells, *Neurosci. Lett. 151*, 146–149.

49. Waksman, M., Eli, Y., Liscovitch, M., and Gerst, J.E. (1996) Identification and Characterization of a Gene Encoding Phospholipase D Activity in Yeast, *J. Biol. Chem. 271*, 2361–2364.

50. Ktistakis, N.T., Brown, H.A., Waters, M.G., Sternweis, P.C., and Roth, M.G. (1996) Evidence That Phospholipase D Mediates ADP Ribosylation Factor-Dependent Formation of Golgi Coated Vesicles, *J. Cell Biol. 134*, 295–306.

51. Liscovitch, M., and Cantley. L.C. (1995) Signal Transduction and Membrane Traffic: The PITP/Phosphoinositide Connection. *Cell 81*, 659–662.
52. De Camilli, P., Emr, S.D., McPherson. P.S., and Novick, P. (1996) Phosphoinositides as Regulators in Membrane Traffic. *Science 271*, 1533–1539.
53. Wang, X., Xu, L., and Zheng. L. (1994) Cloning and Expression of Phosphatidylcholine-Hydrolyzing Phospholipase D from *Ricinus communis* L., *J. Biol. Chem. 269*, 20312–20317.
54. Rose, K., Rudge, S.A., Frohman, M.A., Morris, A.J., and Engebrecht, J. (1995) Phospholipase D Signaling is Essential for Meiosis, *Proc. Natl. Acad. Sci. USA 92*, 12151–12155.
55. Ella, K., Dolan, J.W., Qi, C., and Meier. K.E. (1996) Characterization of *Saccharomyces cerevisiae* Deficient in Expression of Phospholipase D, *Biochem. J. 314*, 15–19.
56. Hammond, S.M., Altshuller, Y.M., Sung. T.-C., Rudge, S.A., Rose, K., Engebrecht, J., Morris, A.J., and Frohman, M.A. (1995) Human ADP-Ribosylation Factor-Activated Phosphatidylcholine-Specific Phospholipase D Defines a New and Highly Conserved Gene Family, *J. Biol. Chem. 270*, 29640–29643.
57. Mayr, J.A., Kohlwein, S.D., and Paltauf, F. (1996) Identification of a Novel, Ca^{2+}-Dependent Phospholipase D with Preference for Phosphatidylserine and Phosphatidylethanolamine in *Saccharomyces cervisiae*, *FEBS Lett. 393*, 236–240.
58. Waksman, M., Tang, X., Eli, Y., Gerst, J.E., and Liscovitch, M. (1997) Identification of a Novel Ca^{2+}-Dependent, Phosphatidylethanolamine-Hydrolyzing Phospholipase D in Yeast Bearing a Disruption in *PLD1*, *J. Biol. Chem. 272*, 36–39.

Chapter 6

Phosphatidylserine as a Signal for Recognition and Phagocytosis: The Proteins Involved

Robert A. Schlegel[a], Stephen Krahling[a], Allison J. Christie[b], and Patrick Williamson[b]

[a]Department of Biochemistry and Molecular Biology, Penn State University, University Park, PA 16802, [b]Department of Biology, Amherst College, Amherst, MA 01002

Transbilayer Phospholipid Asymmetry

When phospholipids form bilayers *in vitro*, different species of phospholipids randomly assort between the two leaflets of the bilayer, at least in the absence of imposed physicochemical gradients. However, in the plasma membranes of all eukaryotic cells thus far examined, and in some internal transport vesicles as well, the phospholipids are not symmetrically distributed across the bilayer. Rather, the bilayer is arranged such that the choline phospholipids predominate in the extracytosolic leaflet and the aminophospholipids predominate in the cytosolic leaflet (1). Several proteins have been identified that are responsible for maintaining or dissipating this asymmetric transbilayer distribution, and others that mediate the physiological consequences of alterations in this distribution have also been identified.

Measuring Lipid Distributions

Understanding lipid asymmetry depends on the availability of methods for assessing the transbilayer distribution or movement of phospholipids (Table 6.1). Which method is appropriate in any particular instance depends on the cell type examined and the specific information sought (2). All the methods depend on the application of impermeant reagents to cells or isolated vesicles; phospholipids that are affected by the reagents are thereby shown to reside in the outer leaflet. If the membrane to which the reagents are exposed is the only membrane in the system under analysis, as is the case with erythrocytes (which contain only a plasma membrane) or isolated vesicles, this information is sufficient to establish the transbilayer distribution of phospholipids. However, if there are internal membranes to which the reagents cannot gain access, as is the case for most eukaryotic cells, then unaffected phospholipids include both those in the inner leaflet of the plasma membrane and all lipids from internal membranes. Under these circumstances, the transbilayer distribution of phospholipids in the plasma membrane generally cannot be established. Even so, the assays can quantify phospholipids (or their analogs) in the outer leaflet.

TABLE 6.1
Methods for Measuring Transbilayer Distribution of Phospholipids

	Reagents	Advantages	Disadvantages	References
Biochemical modification	Phospholipases Trinitrobenzenesulfonic acid Fluorescamine	Direct	Laborious, problematic with complex cells, only populations	2
Fluorescence	MC540	Simple, single-cell	Indirect, proven only with blood cells	3–8,29
	Fluoresceinated annexin	Simple, single-cell	Measures only PS, semi-quantitative	11
	Fluorescent phospholipids (translocase/scramblase assays)	Simple, single-cell	Distribution inferred	12,15,30
Radioactive	Iodinated annexin	Quantitative	Measures only PS, only populations	10
Procoagulant	Clotting assay reagents	Physiologically relevant		5,9,31

In erythrocytes the two leaflets of the plasma membrane differ in their physical properties. Loss of phospholipid asymmetry results in loss of these differences, thereby changing the physical properties of the outer leaflet. Detecting changes in one of these physical properties forms the basis of an indirect assay of asymmetry. The phospholipids in the outer leaflet of the erythrocyte membrane are tightly packed and largely exclude the impermeant lipophilic fluorophore merocyanine 540 (MC540). On loss of asymmetry the packing of the outer leaflet becomes looser as phospholipids from the inner leaflet are introduced into it, and binding of MC540 is enhanced. Thus, measurement of MC540 binding can be used to determine whether erythrocytes maintain or lose asymmetry after various treatments (3,4). Given that the composition and distribution of phospholipids in the plasma membranes of other blood cells are similar to those of erythrocytes (1), MC540 staining has also been used to identify lymphocytes (5–7) and neutrophils (8) that have lost their asymmetry.

As the aminophospholipid phosphatidylserine (PS) resides exclusively in the inner leaflet of blood cells, its appearance on the cell surface has been taken as an indication of loss of asymmetry. Two methods, based on specific recognition of PS by proteins, are now commonly used to make such an assessment. The first method exploits the fact that PS exposed on the surface of cells provides binding sites for the assembly of factor complexes VIIIaIXa (tenase) and VaXa (prothrombinase) in the coagulation cascade. Thus, surface-exposed PS can be measured as the procoagulant activity of cells in coagulation assays (9). The second method depends on the use of annexins: proteins that specifically bind PS in the presence of Ca^{2+}. Annexins labeled with a radioactive (10) or fluorescent (11) tag can be used to measure surface-exposed PS. These two assays assume that the appearance of PS on the cell surface denotes loss of phospholipid asymmetry, even though the distribution of only one lipid species—PS—is being measured. It is also often assumed that PS is reaching the surface from the inner leaflet of the plasma membrane and not by some other mechanism, such as addition of new membrane to the plasma membrane during exocytosis.

While these assays are invaluable in establishing the equilibrium distribution of phospholipids, insight into how these distributions come about and their underlying dynamics has come from assays that measure transbilayer movement of phospholipids. Such assays reveal the existence of two membrane activities that govern the distribution of phospholipids and that also serve to illustrate the assays that detect them.

The Aminophospholipid Translocase

Because phospholipids diffuse passively across biological membranes over the course of several hours, the persistence of a nonrandom distribution of phospholipids immediately implies an active process at work. In fact, the plasma membranes of every cell thus far examined, from erythrocytes to fibroblasts to sperm, and the membranes of some internal transport vesicles as well, all contain an ATP-dependent activity that specifically transports aminophospholipids from the extracytosolic to the cytosolic side of the membrane (Fig. 6.1).

This translocase activity is revealed in assays of transbilayer lipid movement such as the one presented in Fig. 6.2. Fluorescent phospholipid analogs were introduced into the outer leaflet of the plasma membrane of *T* lymphocyte hybridoma

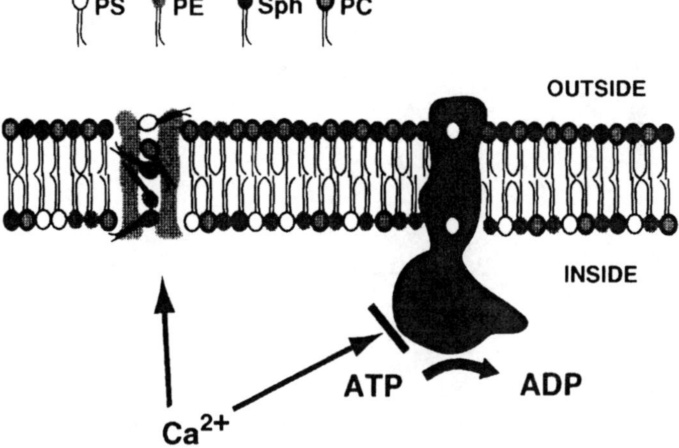

Fig. 6.1. Proteins that regulate transbilayer distribution of phospholipids. At left, the scramblase is activated by Ca^{2+}; at right, the ATP-dependent aminophospholipid translocase is inactivated by Ca^{2+}. Aminophospholipids include phosphatidylserine (PS) and phosphatidylethanolamine (PE); choline phospholipids include phosphatidylcholine (PC) and sphingomyelin (Sph).

cells. After a 10 min incubation to allow transport, dithionite was added to a concentration that reduced all external probe within 30 s, and fluorescence was recorded continuously. The difference in fluorescence at 30 s between cells labeled with an analog of PS and cells labeled with an analog of the zwitterion phosphatidylcholine (PC) represents PS internalized by the translocase and thereby inaccessible to reduc-

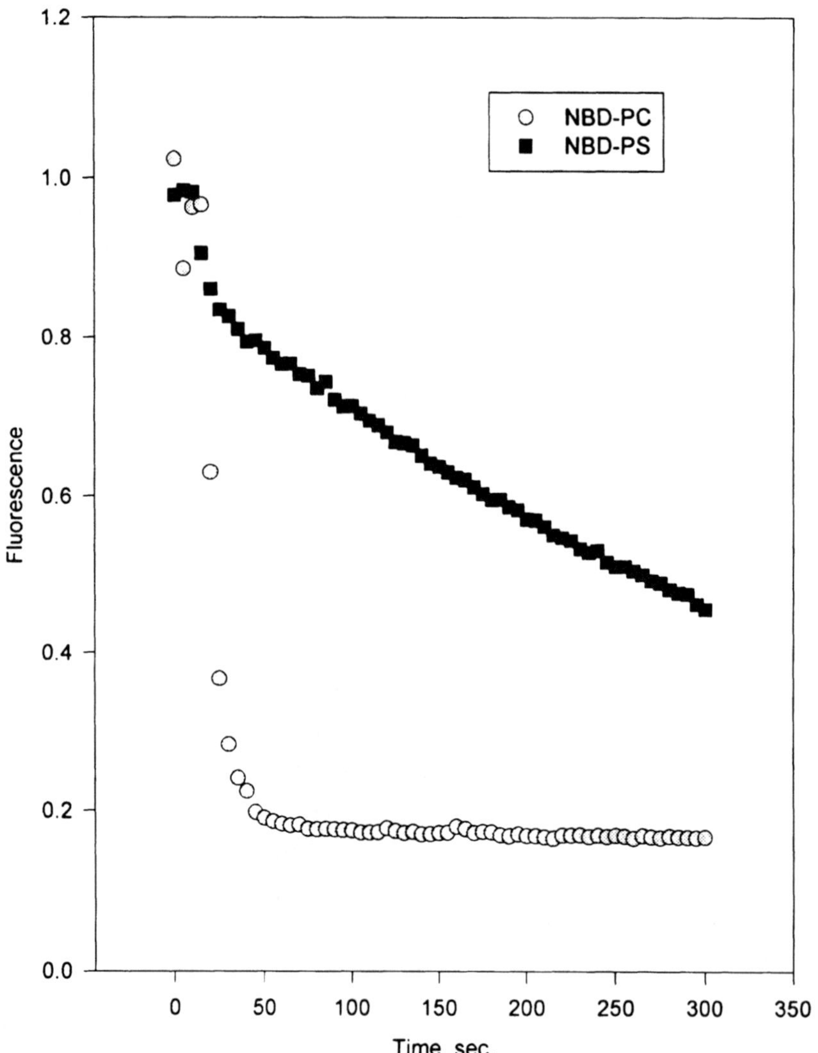

Fig. 6.2. Measuring translocase activity. DO11.10 *T* lymphocyte hybridoma cells were incubated at 37°C for 10 min in the presence of PS or PC labeled with 7-nitro-2,1,3-benzoxadiazol-4-yl (NBD). The cells were then transferred to a fluorimeter, 2 mM sodium dithionite added, and fluorescence recorded continuously.

tion by dithionite (12). Subsequent changes in fluorescence represent the transbilayer movement of internalized probe to the cell surface *via* passive diffusion, where it is reduced by dithionite. The search for the ATP-dependent aminophospholipid translocase responsible for the transport has been intense since its initial discovery in 1984 (13), and several candidate proteins have been identified (Table 6.2).

Using photoactivable analogs of PS, Schroit and colleagues identified a 32-kD protein that was specifically labeled when the probe was applied to erythrocytes (14). The same protein was labeled by a potent inhibitor of the translocase (15,16), leading to the suggestion that the protein was the translocase. Monoclonal antibody to the Rhesus (Rh) antigen of erythrocytes immunoprecipitates the 32 kD protein-labeled by both of the probes (17). However, the protein has not been reported as having ATPase activity, nor has it been reconstituted into vesicles and shown to have translocase activity. Further discussion of the 32-kD protein can be found in Diaz and Schroit (18).

ATP-dependent, aminophospholipid-specific translocation has been demonstrated in vesicles into which a 110-kD Mg^{2+} ATPase, purified from erythrocytes, was reconstituted (19). The gene coding for a similar enzyme, the ATPase II of chromaffin granules, has recently been cloned (20). This P-type ATPase shows a striking resemblance to the predicted protein product of the *DRS2* gene of the yeast *Saccharomyces cerevisiae* (21). Although wild-type yeast can efficiently and specifically translocate PS analogs across the plasma membrane, a *drs2* deletion mutant cannot (20), suggesting that the yeast protein, like the ATPase II, is in fact an aminophospholipid translocase. It is now clear that the *DRS2* gene and the gene encoding the mammalian ATPase II are members of a previously unrecognized subfamily of P-type ATPases. The existence of several identifiable classes of genes within this new subfamily suggests that transporters with specificity for other phospholipids or lipid-like molecules may await characterization.

The Scramblase

As indicated in Fig. 6.1, Ca^{2+} inactivates the aminophospholipid translocase (22). However, inactivation of the translocase does not result in the immediate appearance of aminophospholipids on the cell surface, because passive diffusion of phospho-

TABLE 6.2
Candidates for the Aminophospholipid Translocase

	Molecular weight (kD)	Identification	Translocase activity reconstituted	Ref.
Rh protein	32	Photoaffinity labeling	No	14–18
ATPase II/*drs2*/ Mg^{2+} ATPase	130[a]	ATPase activity	Yes[b]	19–21

[a]Calculated from predicted protein product of ATPase II gene.
[b]Erythrocyte Mg^{2+} ATPase only.

lipids across the bilayer requires several hours. However, Ca^{2+} can also induce a rapid bidirectional movement of phospholipids across the bilayer that is nonspecific for lipid type (Fig. 6.1). Thus this activity, termed the scramblase, acts to randomize transbilayer distribution in minutes (23).

Scramblase activity is revealed in assays of transbilayer lipid movement such as the one presented in Fig. 6.3. A fluorescent analog of PS was internalized by *T* lymphocyte hybridoma cells as in Fig. 6.2, dithionite was added to reduce external probe, and fluorescence was recorded continuously. The slow rate of reduction of fluorescence represents return of the probe to the surface *via* passive diffusion, where it is reduced by dithionite. Elevation of cytosolic Ca^{2+} by external addition of Ca^{2+} in the presence of ionophore results in a rapid decrease in fluorescence as the scramblase is activated.

Over the past few years, several candidates for the scramblase have been identified (Table 6.3). One such candidate is not a protein. Rather, it was suggested that an influx of Ca^{2+} into cells might result in the formation of a complex between Ca^{2+} and phosphatidylinositol 4,5-bisphosphate (PIP_2) (24), and that this complex could catalyze transbilayer lipid movements. A second candidate is a protein labeled by a photoactivable phospholipid analog applied to erythrocytes and identified as the 31-kD membrane protein stomatin (25). Interestingly, the same inhibitor of the translocase mentioned above labeled stomatin, leading the authors to suggest that stomatin rather than the Rh protein is the predominant protein labeled by the reagent and that stomatin may be the scramblase (and not the translocase).

The most direct approach to identify and purify the scramblase has been to reconstitute and assay its activity in artificial vesicles. In platelets, this approach resulted in a protein fraction containing three predominant proteins between 20 and 50 kD (26). From erythrocytes, a protein has been purified to apparent homogeneity, with a molecular weight of approximately 37 kD (27). In both cases, reconstitution yielded a Ca^{2+}-dependent, nonspecific, bidirectional movement of phospholipids. Significantly, in both instances the presence of PIP_2 in the reconstitutes had no effect on scramblase activity.

Consequences of Surface-Exposed PS

To date, the most dramatic consequences of loss of membrane asymmetry are ascribable to the appearance of PS on the cell surface. When platelets are activated, the translocase is inhibited, the scramblase is activated, lipid asymmetry is abolished, and PS appears on the platelet surface, as detected by biochemical assays (28), increased MC540 staining (29), and transport assays (30). This sequence of events is a critical step in the pathway leading to blood coagulation (31).

Erythrocytes in which lipid asymmetry is disrupted are more readily phagocytosed by macrophages *in vitro* than are erythrocytes with asymmetric membranes (32). PS vesicles are able to inhibit the increased uptake completely (33), indicating that exposure of PS is the signal by which the erythrocytes are recognized. PS also serves as a

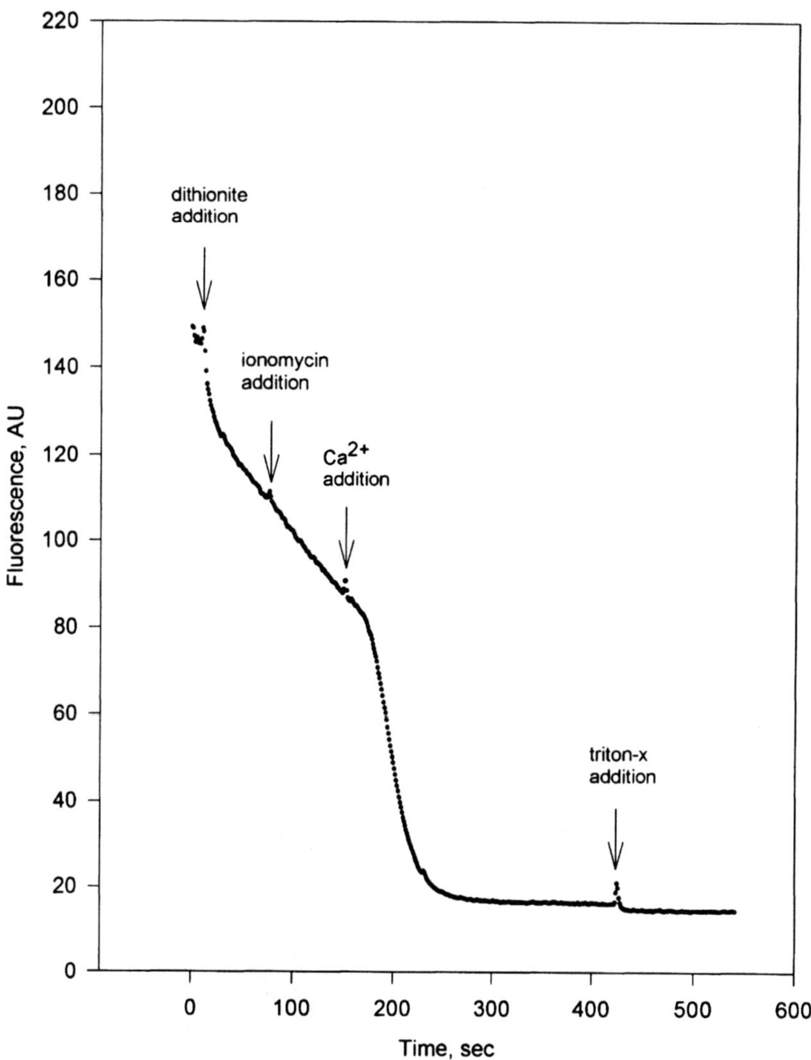

Fig. 6.3. Measuring activation of scramblase activity by Ca^{2+}. DO11.10 cells were labeled with NBD-PS as in Fig. 6.2 and fluorescence continuously recorded during the subsequent addition of 2 mM dithionite, the calcium ionophore ionomycin, 667 µM Ca^{2+}, and finally Triton X-100, which lysed the cells, exposing internal NBD-PS to reduction by dithionite.

recognition signal *in vivo*; when PS is incorporated into artificial lipid vesicles that otherwise resemble the erythrocyte surface, the vesicles are prematurely cleared from the circulation (34). These results suggest that erythrocytes may expose PS on their surface at the end of their normal lifespan as a signal for clearance by macrophages.

TABLE 6.3
Candidates for the Scramblase

	Molecular weight (kD)	Identification	Reference
Ca^{2+}/PIP_2[a]	1	Supplementation	24
Stomatin	31	Photoaffinity labeling	25
Platelet proteins	20–50	Reconstitution	26
Erythrocyte protein	37	Reconstitution	27

[a]PIP_2, phosphatidylinositol 4-5 bisphosphate.

Apoptotic cells are recognized by macrophages and phagocytosed while still intact, preventing inflammation. Lymphocytes undergoing apoptosis down-regulate the translocase, activate the scramblase, and express PS on their surface as part of the apoptotic program, as detected by coagulation assays (5), increased MC540 staining (5–7), increased annexin binding (11, 35) and transport assays (36). It is this PS exposure that provokes their recognition and phagocytosis; enhanced phagocytosis of apoptotic cells can be inhibited by PS vesicles (5), as shown in Fig. 6.4.

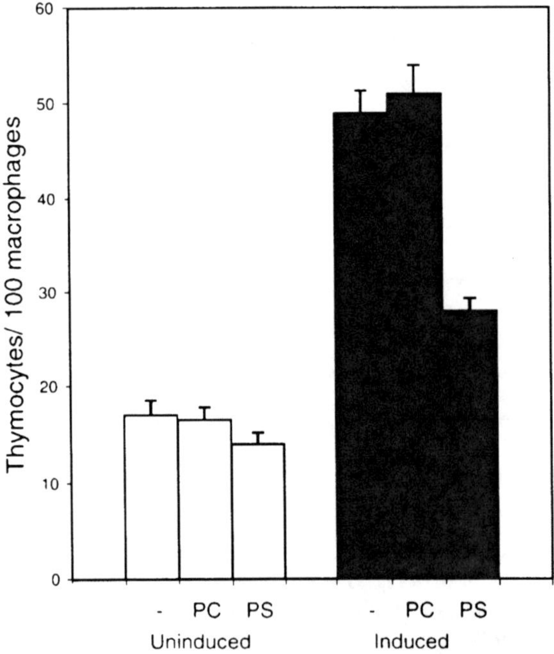

Fig. 6.4. Inhibition of phagocytosis of apoptotic lymphocytes by PS vesicles. Mouse thymocytes were incubated in the presence or absence of 10^{-6} M dexamethasone for 6 h at 37°C to induce apoptosis; mixed with PS, PC, or no vesicles; added to monolayers of elicited mouse peritoneal macrophages; and the number of thymocytes phagocytosed in 30 min counted.

TABLE 6.4
Candidates for PS Receptors

	Molecular weight (kD)	Identification	References
Class B scavenger receptors		PS binding to transfected cells	39
CD36	88 (apparent)		
BI	Unknown		
Macrosialin (CD68)	94–97	PS binding to protein blots	40,41
Protein recognized by monoclonal antibody 61D3	75	Inhibits binding of apoptotic cells by macrophages	42–44,[a]

[a]Pradhan, D., Krahling, S., Williamson, P., and Schlegel, R.A., submitted for publication.

The recognition of apoptotic lymphocytes is, however, far more complex than it is for erythrocytes. First, inhibition by PS vesicles is only partial. Second, uptake of apoptotic cells by some types of macrophages cannot be inhibited by PS vesicles but can be blocked by the tetrapeptide RGDS, implicating an integrin in recognition (37). However, these macrophages can recognize PS, and PS on the surface of erythrocytes can block uptake of apoptotic cells, even though PS in the form of vesicles cannot (Pradhan, D., Krahling, S., Williamson, P., and Schlegel, R.A., submitted for publication). Significantly, PS involvement in the recognition and phagocytosis of apoptotic cells is not restricted to blood cells; normal vascular smooth-muscle cells appear to recognize and phagocytose apoptotic smooth muscle cells at least in part by surface exposure of PS (38).

Regardless of the complexity of recognition of lymphocytes, it is clear that all macrophages are capable of specifically recognizing PS and therefore must have receptors with such specificity. Recently, several different receptors present on macrophages have been implicated in PS recognition (Table 6.4). It will be intriguing to learn which of these or combinations thereof are responsible for the spectrum of PS recognition by macrophages.

Acknowledgments

This research was supported by grants from the American Heart Association, Pennsylvania Affiliate, and the United States National Science Foundation. We thank Margaret S. Halleck for providing Fig. 6.1.

References

1. Williamson, P., and Schlegel, R.A. (1994) Back and Forth: the Regulation and Function of Transbilayer Phospholipid Movement in Eukaryotic Cells (Review), *Molec. Memb. Biol. 11*, 199–216.
2. Roelofsen, B., and Op den Kamp, J.A.F. (1994) Plasma Membrane Phospholipid Asymmetry and Its Maintenance: The Human Erythrocyte as a Model, *Curr. Topics Memb. 40*, 7–46.

3. Schlegel, R.A., Reed, J., McEvoy, L., Algarin, L., and Williamson, P. (1987) Phospholipid Asymmetry of Loaded Red Cells, *Meths. Enzymol. 149*, 293–300.

4. Verhoven, B., Schlegel, R.A., and Williamson, P. (1992) Rapid Loss and Restoration of Lipid Asymmetry by Different Pathways in Resealed Erythrocyte Ghosts, *Biochim. Biophys. Acta 1104*, 15–23.

5. Fadok, V.A., Voelker, D.R., Campbell, P.A., Cohen, J.J., Bratton, D.L., and Henson, P.M. (1992) Exposure of Phosphatidylserine on the Surface of Apoptotic Lymphocytes Triggers Specific Recognition and Removal by Macrophages, *J. Immunol. 148*, 2207–2216.

6. Schlegel, R.A., Stevens, M., Lumley-Sapanski, L., Williamson, P. (1993) Altered Lipid Packing Identifies Apoptotic Thymocytes, *Immunol. Lett. 36*, 283–288.

7. Mower, D.A., Jr., Peckman, D.W., Illera, V.A., Fishaugh, J.K., Stunz, L.L., and Ashman, R.F. (1994) Decreased Membrane Phospholipid Packing and Decreased Cell Size Precede DNA Cleavage in Mature Mouse B Cell Apoptosis, *J. Immunol. 152*, 4832–4842.

8. McEvoy, L., Schlegel, R.A., Williamson, P., and Del Buono, B.J. (1988) Merocyanine 540 as a Flow Cytometric Probe of Membrane Lipid Organization in Leukocytes, *J. Leuk. Biol. 44*, 337–344.

9. Connor, J., Bucana, C., Fidler, I., and Schroit, A.J. (1980) Differentiation-Dependent Expression of Phosphatidylserine in Mammalian Plasma Membranes: Quantitative Assessment of Outer-Leaflet Lipid by Prothrombinase Complex Formation, *Proc. Natl. Acad. Sci. USA 86*, 3184–3188.

10. Thiagarajan, P., and Tait, J.F. (1991) Binding of Annexin V/Placental Anticoagulant Protein I to Platelets: Evidence for Phosphatidylserine Exposure in the Procoagulant Response of Activated Platelets, *J. Biol. Chem. 266*, 24302–24307.

11. Koopman, G., Reutelingsperger, C.P.M., Kuijten, G.A.M., Keehnen, R.M.J., Pals, S.T., and van Oers, M.H.J. (1994) Annexin V for Flow Cytometric Detection of Phosphatidylserine Expression on B Cells Undergoing Apoptosis, *Blood 84*, 1415–1420.

12. McIntyre, J.C., and Sleight, R.G. (1991) Fluorescent Assay for Phospholipid Membrane Asymmetry, *Biochemistry 30*, 11819–11827.

13. Seigneuret, M., and Devaux, P. (1984) ATP-Dependent Asymmetric Distribution of Spin-Labeled Phospholipids in the Erythrocyte Membrane: Relation to Shape Change, *Proc. Natl. Acad. Sci. USA 81*, 3751–3755.

14. Schroit, A.J., Madsen, J., and Ruoho, A.E. (1987) Radioiodinated, Photoactivatable Phosphatidylcholine and Phosphatidylserine: Transfer Properties and Differential Photoreactive Interaction with Human Erythrocyte Membrane Proteins, *Biochemistry 26*, 1812–1819.

15. Connor, J., and Schroit, A.J. (1988) Transbilayer Movement of Phosphatidylserine in Erythrocytes: Inhibition of Transport and Preferential Labeling of a 31000-Dalton Protein by Sulfhydryl Reactive Reagents, *Biochemistry 27*, 848–851.

16. Connor, J., and Schroit, A.J. (1991) Transbilayer Movement of Phosphatidylserine in Erythrocytes. Inhibitors of Aminophospholipid Transport Block the Association of Photolabeled Lipid to Its Transporter, *Biochim. Biophys. Acta 1066*, 37–42.

17. Schroit, A.J., Bloy, C., Connor, J., and Cartron, J.-P. (1990) Involvement of Rh Blood Group Polypeptides in the Maintenance of Aminophospholipid Asymmetry, *Biochemistry 29*, 10303–10306.

18. Diaz, C., and Schroit, A.J. (1996) Role of Translocases in the Generation of Phosphatidylserine Asymmetry, *J. Memb. Biol. 151*, 1–9.

19. Auland, M.E., Roufogalis, B.D., Devaux, P.F., and Zachowski, A. (1994) Reconstitution of ATP-Dependent Aminophospholipid Translocation in Proteoliposomes, *Proc. Natl. Acad. Sci. USA 91*, 10938–10942.

20. Tang, X., Halleck, M.S., Schlegel, R.A., and Williamson, P. (1996) A Subfamily of P-type ATPases with Aminophospholipid Transporting Activity, *Science 272*, 1495–1497.

21. Ripmaster, T.L., Vaughn, G.P., and Woolford, J.L., Jr. (1993) *DRS1* to *DRS7*, Novel Genes Required for Ribosome Assembly and Function in *Saccharomyces cerevisiae*, *Mol. Cell. Biol. 13*, 7901–7912.

22. Bitbol, M., Fellmann, P., Zachowski, A., and Devaux, P.F. (1987) Ion Regulation of Phosphatidylserine and Phosphatidylethanolamine Outside-Inside Translocation in Human Erythrocytes, *Biochim. Biophys. Acta 904*, 268–282.

23. Williamson, P., Kulick, A., Zachowski, A., Schlegel, R.A., and Devaux, P.F. (1992) Ca^{++} Induces Transbilayer Redistribution of All Major Phospholipids in Human Erythrocytes, *Biochemistry 31*, 6355–6360.

24. Sulpice, J.-C., Zachowski, A., Devaux, P.F., and Giraud, F. (1994) Requirement for Phosphatidylinositol 4,5-bisphosphate in the Ca^{2+}-Induced Phospholipid Redistribution in the Human Erythrocyte Membrane, *J. Biol. Chem. 269*, 6347–6354.

25. Desneves, J., Berman, A., Dynon, K., La Greca, N., Foley, M., and Tilley, L. (1996) Human Erythrocyte Band 7.2b Is Preferentially Labeled by a Photoreactive Phospholipid, *Biochem. Biophys. Res. Commun. 224*, 108–114.

26. Comfurius, P., Williamson, P., Smeets, E.F., Schlegel, R.A., Bevers, E.M., and Zwaal, R.F.A. (1996) Reconstitution of Phospholipid Scramblase Activity from Human Blood Platelets, *Biochemistry 35*, 7631–7634.

27. Basse, F., Stout, J.G., Sims, P.J., and Wiedmer, T. (1996) Isolation of an Erythrocyte Membrane Protein That Mediates Ca^{2+}-Dependent Transbilayer Movement of Phospholipid, *J. Biol. Chem. 271*, 17205–17210.

28. Bevers, E.M., Comfurius, P., and Zwaal, R.F.A. (1983) Changes in Membrane Phospholipid Distribution During Platelet Activation, *Biochim. Biophys. Acta 736*, 57–66.

29. Lupu, F., Calb, M., Scurei, C., and Simionescu, N. (1986) Changes in the Organization of Membrane Lipids During Human Platelet Activation. Study by Fluorescence and Freeze-Fracture Cytochemistry, *Lab. Invest. 54*, 136–145.

30. Williamson, P., Bevers, E.M., Smeets, E.F., Comfurius, P., Schlegel, R.A., and Zwaal, R.F.A. (1995) Continuous Analysis of the Mechanism of Activated Transbilayer Lipid Movement in Platelets, *Biochemistry 34*, 10448–10455.

31. Bevers, E., Comfurius, E.P., Van Rijn, J., Hemker, C., and Zwaal, R.F.A. (1982) Generation of Prothrombin-Converting Activity and the Exposure of Phosphatidylserine at the Outer Surface of Platelets, *Europ. J. Biochem. 122*, 429–436.

32. McEvoy, L., Williamson, P., and Schlegel, R.A. (1986) Membrane Phospholipid Asymmetry as a Determinant of Erythrocyte Recognition by Macrophages, *Proc. Natl. Acad. Sci. USA 83*, 3311–3315.

33. Pradhan, D., Williamson, P., and Schlegel, R.A. (1994) Phosphatidylserine Vesicles Inhibit Phagocytosis of Erythrocytes with a Symmetric Distribution of Phospholipids, *Molec. Memb. Biol. 11*, 181–188.

34. Allen, T.M., Williamson, P., and Schlegel, R.A. (1988) Phosphatidylserine as a Determinant of Reticuloendothelial Recognition of Liposome Models of the Erythrocyte Surface, *Proc. Natl. Acad. Sci. USA 85*, 8067–8071.

35. Martin, S.J., Reutelingsperger, C.P.M., McGahon, A.J., Rader, J.A., van Schie,

R.C.A.A., LaFace, D.M., and Green, D.R. (1995) Early Redistribution of Plasma Membrane Phosphatidylserine Is a General Feature of Apoptosis Regardless of the Initiating Stimulus: Inhibition by Overexpression of Bcl-2 and Abl, *J. Exp. Med. 182*, 1545–1556.

36. Verhoven, B., Schlegel, R.A., and Williamson, P. (1995) Mechanisms of Phosphatidylserine Exposure, a Phagocytic Recognition Signal, on Apoptotic T Lymphocytes, *J. Exp. Med. 182*, 1597–1601.

37. Fadok, V.A., Savill, J.S., Haslett, C., Bratton, D.L., Doherty, D.E., Campbell, P., and Henson, P.M. (1992) Different Populations of Macrophages Use Either the Vitronectin Receptor or the Phosphatidylserine Receptor to Recognize and Remove Apoptotic Cells, *J. Immunol. 149*, 4029–4035.

38. Bennett, M.R., Gibson, D.F., Schwartz, S.M., and Tait, J.F. (1995) Binding and Phagocytosis of Apoptotic Vascular Smooth Muscle Cells Is Mediated in Part by Exposure of Phosphatidylserine, *Circ. Res. 77*, 1136–1142.

39. Rigotti, A., Acton, S.L., and Krieger, M. (1995) The Class B Scavenger Receptors SR-BI and CD36 Are Receptors for Anionic Phospholipids, *J. Biol. Chem. 270*, 16221–16224.

40. Sambrano, G.R., and Steinberg, D. (1995) Recognition of Oxidatively Damaged and Apoptotic Cells by an Oxidized Low Density Lipoprotein Receptor on Mouse Peritoneal Macrophages: Role of Membrane Phosphatidylserine, *Proc. Natl. Acad. Sci. USA 92*, 1396–1400.

41. Ramprasad, M.P., Fischer, W., Witztum, J.L., Sambrano, G.R., Quehenberger, O., and Steinberg, D. (1995) The 94- to 97-kDa Mouse Macrophage Membrane Protein That Recognizes Oxidized Low Density Lipoprotein and Phosphatidylserine-Rich Liposomes Is Identical to Macrosialin, the Mouse Homologue of Human CD68, *Proc. Natl. Acad. Sci. USA 92*, 9580–9584.

42. Ugolini, V., Nunez, G., Smith, R.G., Stastny, P., and Capra, J.D. (1980) Initial Characterization of Monoclonal Antibodies against Human Monocytes, *Proc. Natl. Acad. Sci. USA 77*, 6764–6768.

43. Nunez, G., Ugolini, V., Capra, J.D., and Stastny, P. (1982) Monoclonal Antibodies Against Human Monocytes. II. Recognition of Two Distinct Cell Surface Molecules, *Scand. J. Immunol. 16*, 515–523.

44. Flora, P.K., and Gregory, C.D. (1994) Recognition of Apoptotic Cells by Human Macrophages: Inhibition by a Monocyte/Macrophage-Specific Monoclonal Antibody, *Europ. J. Immunol. 24*, 2625–2632.

Chapter 7

Neurochemical Effects of Altered Prenatal Choline Availability in Rats

Jan Krzysztof Blusztajn[a], Thomas Holler[b], Jennifer Marie Cermak[b], and Darrell A. Jackson[b]

[a]Departments of Pathology and Psychiatry, Boston University School of Medicine, Boston, MA 02118, [b]Department of Pathology, Boston University School of Medicine, Boston, MA 02118

Introduction

Over the last two decades a large body of data obtained by workers in various laboratories has shown that choline supplementation (*in vivo* or *in vitro*) increases the levels of the neurotransmitter acetylcholine (ACh) and modulates postsynaptic events consistent with enhanced cholinergic transmission (1–2). Moreover, since cholinergic neurotransmission is important in the physiology of memory, choline has been used as a possible memory-enhancing drug (3). However, in addition to being a precursor for ACh, choline is also required for the synthesis of phosphatidylcholine (PC) and sphingomyelin (two major components of biological membranes), and it is this function of choline that makes it essential for the growth and survival of mammalian cells (4). In the brain, cell division and rapid membrane synthesis occur primarily during the prenatal and early postnatal periods; thus, choline availability might be especially important for the developing brain. This rationale proved successful in the studies of Meck and Williams and their colleagues, who showed that dietary choline supplementation in pregnant rats resulted in improved performance of the offspring in memory tests (5–7).

The molecular mechanisms by which choline administration to pregnant rats leads to a permanent improvement in memory of the offspring are unknown, but they may include alterations of ACh synthesis and release (1) or be related to the function of choline-containing phospholipids in cell signaling events in the brain (8).

We have tested both of those possibilities by measuring indices of cholinergic function and PC turnover in the hippocampus, a brain region important for the processes of visuospatial memory (9,10). As markers of ACh turnover, we used the activities of choline acetyltransferase (ChAT) and acetylcholinesterase (AChE) as well as the rate of incorporation of [^{14}C]choline into [^{14}C]ACh. As an index of PC turnover, we used the activity of phospholipase D (PLD), a PC-hydrolyzing enzyme that produces phosphatidic acid and choline. Choline formed from PC by PLD can be used for the formation of ACh (11), whereas phosphatidic acid has been implicated as a second messenger in peripheral tissues (12). Furthermore, since phosphatidic acid can be rapidly hydrolyzed by phosphatidic acid phosphohydrolase to 1,2-*sn*-diacylglycerol (DAG), PLD activity contributes to the cellular accumulation of DAG, an activator of protein kinase C (PKC) (13,14). Generation of DAG, and PKC activity, in the hippocampus may be important in the molecular mechanisms of synaptic long-term potentiation—a physiological model for learning and memory in the hippocampus (15). Thus, changes in PLD activity in this brain region may contribute to the changes in memory performance observed after prenatal choline supplementation *in vivo*.

Methods

Prenatal Choline Treatment

Prenatal choline treatments were carried out from day 11 to day 17 of gestation in three groups of pregnant Sprague-Dawley CD-strain rats: supplemented, control, and deficient. The supplemented group received AIN-76A diet, containing 7.9 mmol/kg choline chloride (Dyets Inc., Bethlehem, PA), and water *ad libitum*, containing 25 mM choline chloride and sweetened with 50 mM saccharin, resulting in an average daily choline intake of 4.6 mmol/kg/day. Controls received AIN-76A diet, containing 7.9 mmol/kg choline chloride, and water sweetened with 50 mM saccharin, resulting in an average daily choline intake of 1.3 mmol/kg/day. The deficient group received AIN-76A diet that contained no choline, and water sweetened with 50 mM saccharin. No significant differences in the amounts of diet or water consumed by the different groups was observed. After day 17 of gestation, all animals consumed AIN-76A diet containing 7.9 mmol/kg choline chloride and saccharin-free water. After birth, pups were kept together with their mothers until weaning on day 22 and then housed in same-sex pairs.

PLD Activity in Hippocampal Slices

Hippocampal slices (0.4 mm thick) were preincubated at 37°C for 15 min in 5 mL HBS—that is, HEPES (4-(2-hydroxyethyl)-1-piperazineethanesulfonic acid)-buffered saline solution (composition, in mM: NaCl, 145; KCl, 5; $MgSO_4$, 1; $CaCl_2$, 1.8; glucose, 10; HEPES, 10; pH 7.4). Slices were then labeled for 2 h in 5 mL HBS containing 40 µCi of [^{3}H]glycerol (40 µM) or 25 µCi of [^{3}H]oleic acid (0.54 µM). Labeled slices were placed in incubation chambers (approximately 0.5 mg of protein per chamber) containing 2 mL of HBS and incubated for 30 min at 37°C to wash out the unincorporated label.

To determine PLD activity, the formation of labeled phosphatidylpropanol (PP) in the presence of propanol was measured; PP production is catalyzed exclusively by PLD (16) and provides a convenient index of PLD activity. After labeling and washing, slices were incubated for 30 min at 37°C in HBS in the presence or in the absence of 1-propanol (267 mM) with or without additional drugs. The lipids were extracted according to the procedure of Folch et al. (17), aliquots of the lipid phase were dried, and the radioactivity was measured by liquid scintillation counting. PP was separated from the other lipids by thin-layer chromatography, with the upper phase of a mixture of ethyl acetate/isooctane/acetic acid/water (13/2/3/10, by vol.) as mobile phase. Spots comigrating with PP standards were scraped off the chromatography plates; their radioactivity was measured by liquid scintillation counting and expressed as a percentage of the radioactivity present in the total lipids.

$[^{14}C]ACh$ Synthesis in Hippocampal Slices

Hippocampal slices (obtained as above) were preincubated in HBS/neostigmine (HBS containing 0.1 mM neostigmine) at 37°C for 2 h. Slices were then labeled for 10 min in 2.5 mL HBS/neostigmine containing 1 µM $[^{14}C]$choline. After labeling and washing twice with ice-cold HBS/neostigmine, slices were extracted according to the procedure of Folch et al. (17). $[^{14}C]ACh$ was purified, and its radioactivity and mass were determined by high-performance liquid chromatography (11).

ChAT and AChE Activity in Hippocampal Homogenates

Hippocampi were dissected and kept at –80°C. Homogenates were prepared by sonication in sucrose buffer (composition, in mM: sucrose, 250; HEPES, 10; EDTA, 1; pH 7.2). ChAT activity was determined according to the method of Fonnum (18), and AChE activity was determined by a modification of this method (19).

Results

Prenatal Choline Status and Hippocampal Cholinergic Markers

We measured the activities of the acetylcholine-synthesizing enzyme, ChAT, and of the acetylcholine-degrading enzyme, AChE, in hippocampi of male rats born to mothers exposed to varying amounts of dietary choline during the eleventh (E11) through the seventeenth (E17) day of pregnancy. Prenatal availability of choline affected the development of hippocampal ChAT (Fig. 7.1) and AChE (Fig. 7.2) activity measured on postnatal days (P) 17 and 27. Those activities were highest in the prenatally deficient rats and were lowest in the prenatally supplemented animals. Thus, the postnatal developmental pattern of the two hippocampal cholinergic markers depends on the availability of choline during embryogenesis.

To determine the rate of ACh synthesis in hippocampal slices, we measured the incorporation of radiolabeled $[^{14}C]$choline into $[^{14}C]ACh$. The specific radioactivity of the newly synthesized $[^{14}C]ACh$ depended on prenatal availability of choline (Fig. 7.3). Slices from prenatally deficient animals contained $[^{14}C]ACh$ with the highest specific radioactivity, whereas slices from the prenatally supplemented rats contained $[^{14}C]ACh$ with the lowest specific radioactivity, indicating that the former synthesized the highest fraction of their ACh pool, and the latter the lowest, from the labeled precursor. These data are consistent with the differences in ChAT activities

     J.K. Blusztajn et al.

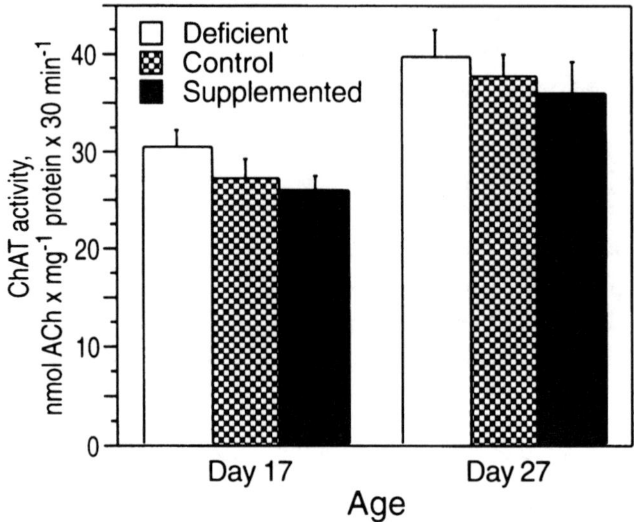

Fig. 7.1. Effect of prenatal availability of choline on choline acetyltransferase activity in rat hippocampus. Male pups at different ages, born to mothers in the deficient, control, and supplemented treatment groups as described in the text, were used for the determination of hippocampal ChAT activity. Statistical analysis by two-way ANOVA indicated a significant effect of choline, $P < 0.01$.

noted above. Moreover, they indicate that the ACh turnover at rest is relatively highest in slices from prenatally deficient rats and the lowest in slices from prenatally supplemented animals.

Prenatal Choline Status and Phospholipase D Activity

Whereas the activities of ChAT and AChE in the hippocampus of prenatally choline-supplemented rats were decreased (Figs. 7.1 and 7.2), hippocampal PLD activity was significantly elevated by this treatment on P7 and P21 (but not P1) (Figs. 7.4 and 7.5). PLD is activated by a variety of neurotransmitter receptors, including the metabotropic glutamate receptor (20). Therefore, the effect of prenatal choline treatments on PLD activity in the presence of glutamate was determined. Consistent with previous findings (20), glutamate (1 mM) increased PLD activity on P7 by 100% in control animals (Fig. 7.5). Choline supplementation increased the glutamate-stimulated component of PLD activity by 35% (Fig. 7.5). Prenatal choline deficiency had no effect on the PLD response to glutamate. Thus, prenatal choline supplementation stimulates both basal and the glutamate-evoked PLD activity in the hippocampus in an age-dependent fashion.

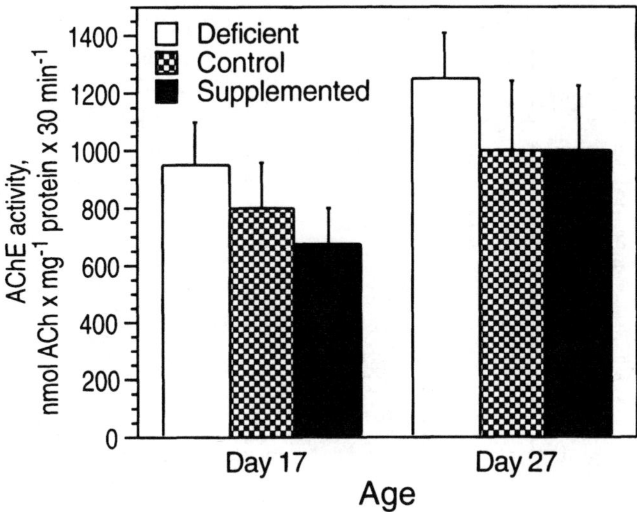

Fig. 7.2. Effect of prenatal availability of choline on acetyl-cholinesterase activity in rat hippocampus. Male pups at different ages, born to mothers in the deficient, control, and supplemented treatment groups as described in the text, were used for the determination of hippocampal AChE activity. Statistical analysis by two-way ANOVA indicated a significant effect of choline, $P < 0.01$.

Discussion

Prenatal choline supplementation during embryonic days 11 through 17 leads to a lifelong improvement of visuospatial memory in rats (5,7). In the present study we report neurochemical sequelae of altered prenatal choline availability during postnatal development. Those include changes in hippocampal ACh turnover and an increase in basal and glutamate-stimulated PLD activity.

The observed cholinergic effects form an interesting pattern of changes. ChAT activity (ACh synthesis) and AChE activity (ACh degradation) are highest in the hippocampus from the prenatally choline-deficient animals and the lowest in the prenatally choline-supplemented ones. Thus, prenatal choline status appears to determine the development of the cholinergic system in the hippocampus; the hippocampal ACh turnover rate in young animals is set by the availability of choline *in utero*. The fast turnover of ACh in the hippocampus of animals deprived of choline during late fetal development may be necessary to enable them to use the available choline more efficiently—that is, to recycle the compound rapidly. The prenatally supplemented animals, on the other hand, presumably have larger reserves of choline and so can "afford" to have a slower ACh turnover. Thus, one would expect that in a prenatally choline-supplemented rat the degradation of intrasynaptic

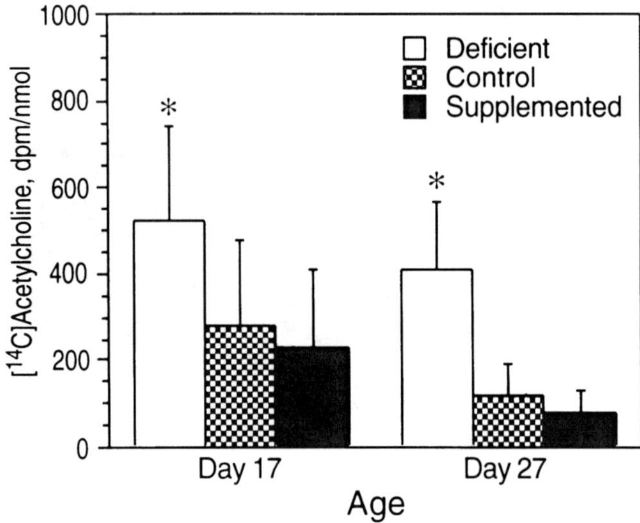

Fig. 7.3. Effect of prenatal choline on [^{14}C]choline incorporation into [^{14}C]ACh in hippocampal slices. Slices from both male and female pups were labeled with [^{14}C]choline and [^{14}C]ACh determined as described in the text. The results are expressed as specific radioactivities. The values from choline-deficient animals were statistically different from the control and from supplemented groups (*$P < 0.03$; Tukey test).

ACh would be slower because of the low AChE activity, resulting in increased cholinergic neurotransmission. Studies. now in progress, are designed to test this hypothesis by determining the effects of prenatal choline availability on muscarinic receptor functioning in the hippocampus.

PLD activity was also altered by choline treatments. Interestingly, the increase in basal PLD activity in hippocampal slices was late in onset (2 weeks after the end of treatment) and long-lasting (until at least 4 weeks after the end of treatment) (see Fig. 4), suggesting an enduring change in hippocampal biochemistry that could contribute to the formation of enhanced memory performance. In intact hippocampal slices, PLD can be activated by numerous G protein–coupled receptors, including α-adrenergic receptors (21). metabotropic glutamate receptors (20,22), and histamine H_1-receptors and endothelin-1 receptors (23), but also by direct stimulation of trimeric G proteins with aluminum fluoride (24) and by stimulation of PKC with phorbol esters (21). We examined the effects of prenatal choline supplementation on stimulated PLD activity in hippocampal slices, using glutamate as an agonist of the glutamatergic receptors. and found that on P7 prenatal choline supplementation increased glutamate-stimulated PLD activity.

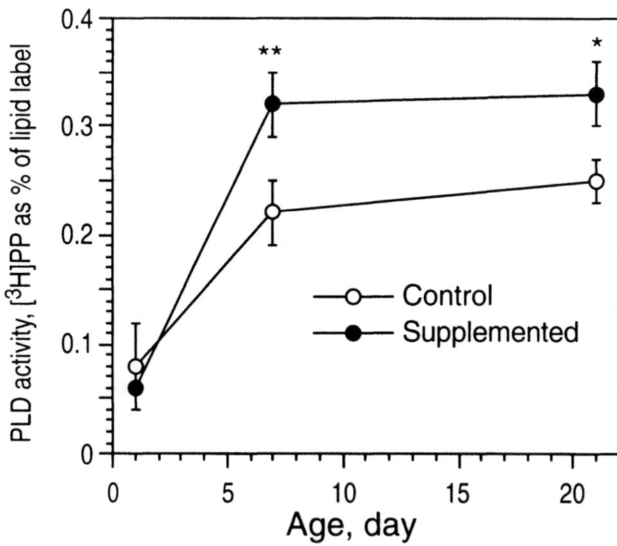

Fig. 7.4. Effect of prenatal choline on the activity of phospholipase D in hippocampal slices. Slices from male pups as in Fig. 7.1 were labeled with [³H]glycerol, washed, and incubated with buffer in the presence of 2% propanol, and radioactivity of the resulting phosphatidylpropanol was determined, as described in the text. The results are expressed as a percentage of the radioactivity in total lipids (*$P < 0.05$ vs. controls; **$P < 0.01$ vs. controls; Fisher's least significant difference test).

Taken together, these results demonstrate that prenatal choline supplementation leads to biochemical changes in the hippocampus. The time course of the effect of prenatal choline supplementation on cholinergic indices and PLD activity correlates with the maturation of the hippocampal formation, which occurs mainly postnatally in the rat (25,26); afferent innervation reaches the hippocampus during the first two weeks after birth (27–30), when many new synapses are formed. This correlation supports the hypothesis that the choline effect on PLD activity is dependent on the presence of an intact hippocampus with its afferent inputs. It is possible that the formation of those inputs is responsible for the fact that the effect of choline could not be detected on P1 but was observed on P7 and P21.

It remains to be determined whether the increase in PLD activity plays a role in the induction and maintenance of memory facilitation in choline-supplemented animals or only accompanies it. Although the physiological functions of PLD in the brain are still poorly understood, the enzyme may be involved in hippocampal synaptic plasticity and memory. Stimulation of metabotropic glutamate receptors in the hippocampus activates PLD and also induces (31) and facilitates (32,33) long-

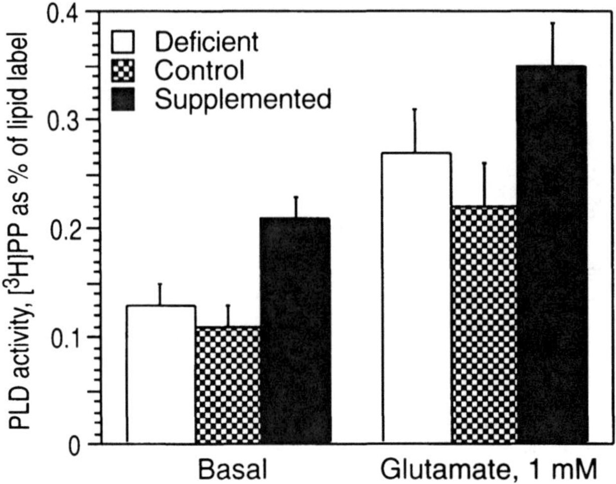

Fig. 7.5. Effect of prenatal choline on basal and glutamate-stimulated activity of phospholipase D in hippocampal slices on P7. Slices from male pups as in Fig. 7.1 were prepared on P7, labeled with [³H]oleate, washed, and incubated with buffer in the presence of 2% propanol in the presence or absence of 1 mM glutamate as described in the text. Radioactivity of the resulting phosphatidylpropanol was determined as described in the text. The results are expressed as a percentage of the radioactivity in total lipids. Statistical analysis by two one-way ANOVAs followed by Fisher's test indicated a significant effect of choline supplementation relative to control ($P < 0.05$).

term potentiation, which is considered a model for learning and memory processes (15). Diacylglycerols (DAG) produced from the PLD-generated phosphatidic acid activate PKC (13), an important step for the maintance of long-term potentiation (34). Moreover, phosphatidylinositol-4,5-bisphosphate and ADP-ribosylation factor, both of which are implicated in membrane trafficking events (35,36), have recently been discovered to activate a membrane-bound PLD (37–39), suggesting a possible role for the enzyme in vesicle trafficking and neurotransmitter release. It is also possible that high PLD activity in rats prenatally supplemented with choline provides more choline for ACh synthesis during times of need, as when the cholinergic hippocampal nerve terminals fire frequently. This is likely to occur when the hippocampus is engaged in solving visuospatial memory tasks.

The demonstration of the influence of prenatal choline status on hippocampal turnover of ACh and on PLD activity and spatial memory performance in the offspring indicate the importance of choline intake during pregnancy for brain development.

Acknowledgments

We thank Ross O. Davis for technical assistance. This work was supported by Grant AG09525 from NIA, National Institutes of Health.

References

1. Blusztajn, J.K., and Wurtman, R.J. (1983) Choline and Cholinergic Neurons, *Science 221*, 614–620.
2. Wecker, L., Cawley, G., and Rothermel, S. (1989) Acute Choline Supplementation In Vivo Enhances Acetylcholine Synthesis In Vitro When Neurotransmitter Release Is Increased by Potassium, *J. Neurochem. 52*, 568–575.
3. Bartus, R.T., Dean, R.L. III, Beer, B., and Lippa, A.S. (1982) The Cholinergic Hypothesis of Geriatric Memory Dysfunction, *Science 217*, 408–417.
4. Eagle, H. (1955) The Minimum Vitamin Requirements of the L and HeLa Cells in Tissue Culture, the Production of Specific Vitamin Deficiencies, and Their Cure, *J. Exp. Med. 102*, 595.
5. Meck, W.H., Smith, R.A., and Williams, C.L. (1988) Pre- and Postnatal Choline Supplementation Produces Long-Term Facilitation of Spatial Memory, *Dev. Psychobiol. 21*, 339–353.
6. Loy, R., Heyer, D., Williams, C.L. and Meck, W.H. (1991) Choline-Induced Spatial Memory Facilitation Correlates with Altered Distribution and Morphology of Septal Neurons, *Adv. Exp. Med. Biol. 295*, 373–382.
7. Meck, W.H., Smith, R.A., and Williams, C.L. (1989) Organizational Changes in Cholinergic Activity and Enhanced Visuospatial Memory as a Function of Choline Administered Prenatally or Postnatally or Both, *Behav. Neurosci. 103*, 1234–1241.
8. Zeisel, S.H., and Blusztajn, J.K. (1994) Choline and Human Nutrition, *Annu. Rev. Nutr. 14*, 269–296.
9. Izquierdo, I. (1975) The Hippocampus and Learning, *Prog. Neurobiol. 5*, 37–75.
10. Shen, Y., Specht, S.M., De Saint Ghislain, I., and Li, R. (1994) The Hippocampus: A Biological Model for Studying Learning and Memory, *Prog. Neurobiol. 44*, 485–496.
11. Lee, H.-C., Fellenz-Maloney, M.-P., Liscovitch, M., and Blusztajn, J.K. (1993) Phospholipase D-Catalyzed Hydrolysis of Phosphatidylcholine Provides the Choline Precursor for Acetylcholine Synthesis in a Human Neuronal Cell Line, *Proc. Natl. Acad. Sci. USA 90*, 10086–10090.
12. Klein, J., Chalifa, V., Liscovitch, M., and Löffelholz, K. (1995) Role of Phospholipase D Activation in Nervous System Physiology and Pathophysiology, *J. Neurochem. 65*, 1445–1455.
13. Nishizuka, Y. (1992) Intracellular Signaling by Hydrolysis of Phospholipids and Activation of Protein Kinase C, *Science 258*, 607–614.
14. Exton, J.H. (1994) Phosphatidylcholine Breakdown and Signal Transduction, *Biochim. Biophys. Acta 1212*, 26–42.
15. Bliss, T.V.P., and Collingridge, G.L. (1993) A Synaptic Model of Memory: Long-Term Potentiation in the Hippocampus, *Nature 361*, 31–39.
16. Pai, J.-K., Siegel, M.I., Egan, R.W., and Billah, M.M. (1988) Phospholipase D Catalyzes Phospholipid Metabolism in Chemotactic Peptide-Stimulated HL-60 Granulocytes, *J. Biol. Chem. 263*, 12472–12477.

17. Folch, J., Lees, M., and Sloane-Stanley, G.A. (1957) A Simple Method for the Isolation and Purification of Total Lipids from Animal Tissues, *J. Biol. Chem. 226*, 497–500.

18. Fonnum, F. (1975) A Rapid Radiochemical Method for the Determination of Choline Acetyltransferase, *J. Neurochem. 24*, 407–409.

19. Zeisel, S.H., Milunsky, A., and Blusztajn, J.K. (1980) Prenatal Diagnosis of Neural Tube Defects. V. The Value of Amniotic Fluid Cholinesterase Studies, *Am. J. Obstet. Gynecol. 137*, 481–485.

20. Holler, T., Cappel, E., Klein, J., and Löffelholz, K. (1993) Glutamate Activates Phospholipase D in Hippocampal Slices of Newborn and Adult Rats, *J. Neurochem. 61*, 1569–1572.

21. Llahi, S., and Fain, J.N. (1992) α_1-Adrenergic Receptor-Mediated Activation of Phospholipase D in Rat Cerebral Cortex, *J. Biol. Chem. 267*, 3679–3685.

22. Boss, V., and Conn, P.J. (1992) Metabotropic Excitatory Amino Acid Receptor Activation Stimulates Phospholipase D in Hippocampal Slices, *J. Neurochem. 59*, 2340–2343.

23. Sarri, E., Picatoste, F., and Claro, E. (1995) Histamine H_1 and Endothelin ET_B Receptors Mediate Phospholipase D Stimulation in Rat Brain Hippocampal Slices, *J. Neurochem. 65*, 837–841.

24. Holler, T., Klein, J., and Löffelholz, K. (1994) Phospholipase C and Phospholipase D Are Independently Activated in Rat Hippocampal Slices, *Biochem. Pharmacol. 47*, 411–414.

25. Minkwitz, H.G., and Holz, L. (1975) The Ontogenetic Development of Pyramidal Neurons in the Hippocampus (CA1) of the Rat, *J. Hirnforsch. 16*, 37–54.

26. Minkwitz, H.G. (1976) [Development of Neuronal Structure in the Hippocampus During Pre- and Post-natal Ontogenesis in the Albino Rat. III. Morphometric Determination of Ontogenetic Changes in Dendrite Structure and Spine Distribution on Pyramidal Neurons (CA1) of the Hippocampus] (in German), *J. Hirnforsch. 17*, 255–275.

27. Loy, R., Lynch, G., and Cotman, C.W. (1977) Development of Afferent Lamination in the Fascia Dentata of the Rat, *Brain Res. 121*, 229–243.

28. Singh, S.C. (1977) The Development of Olfactory and Hippocampal Pathways in the Brain of the Rat, *Anat. Embryol. (Berl). 151*, 183–199.

29. Fricke, R., and Cowan, W.M. (1977) An Autoradiographic Study of the Development of the Entorhinal and Commissural Afferents to the Dentate Gyrus of the Rat, *J. Comp. Neurol. 173*, 231–250.

30. Thal, L.J., Gilbertson, E., Armstrong, D.M. and Gage, F.H. (1992) Development of the Basal Forebrain Cholinergic System: Phenotype Expression Prior to Target Innervation, *Neurobiol. Aging 13*, 67–72.

31. Otani, S., and Ben-Ari, Y. (1991) Metabotropic Receptor-Mediated Long-Term Potentiation in Rat Hippocampal Slices, *Europ. J. Pharmacol. 205*, 325–326.

32. Otani, S., Ben-Ari, Y., and Roisin-Lallemand, M.-P. (1993) Metabotropic Receptor Stimulation Coupled to Weak Tetanus Leads to Long-Term Potentiation and a Rapid Elevation of Cytosolic Protein Kinase C Activity, *Brain Res. 613*, 1–9.

33. Behnisch, T., and Reymann, K.G. (1993) Co-activation of Metabotropic Glutamate and N-methyl-D-Aspartate Receptors Is Involved in Mechanisms of Long-Term Potentiation Maintenance in Rat Hippocampal CA1 Neurons, *Neuroscience 54*, 37–47.

34. Linden, D.J., and Routtenberg, A. (1989) The Role of Protein Kinase C in Long-Term Potentiation: A Testable Model, *Brain Res. Rev. 14*, 279–296.

35. Boman, A.L., and Kahn, R.A. (1995) Arf Proteins: The Membrane Traffic Police? *Trends Biochem. Sci. 20*, 147–150.
36. Liscovitch, M., and Cantley, L.C. (1995) Signal Transduction and Membrane Traffic: The PITP/phosphoinositide connection. *Cell 81*, 659-662.
37. Brown, H.A., Gutowski, S., Moomaw, C.R., Slaughter, C., and Sternweis, P.C. (1993) ADP-Ribosylation Factor, a Small GTP-Dependent Regulatory Protein, Stimulates Phospholipase D Activity, *Cell 75*, 1137–1144.
38. Cockcroft, S., Thomas, G.M.H., Fensome, A., Geny, B., Cunningham, E., Gout, I., Hiles, I., Totty, N.F., Truong, O., and Hsuan, J.J. (1994) Phospholipase D: A Downstream Effector of ARF in Granulocytes, *Science 263*, 523–526.
39. Liscovitch, M., Chalifa, V., Pertile, P., Chen, C.-S., and Cantley, L.C. (1994) Novel Function of Phosphatidylinositol 4,5-Bisphosphate as a Cofactor for Brain Membrane Phospholipase D, *J. Biol. Chem. 269*, 21403–21406.

Chapter 8

Origin of Axonal Lipids in Rat Sympathetic Neurons

Jean E. Vance[a], Elena Posse de Chaves[a], Antonio E. Rusiñol[a], Robert B. Campenot[b], Miguel Bussiere[c], and Dennis E. Vance[c]

[a]Lipid and Lipoprotein Research Group and Department of Medicine, University of Alberta, Edmonton, AB, T6G 2S2, Canada, [b]Departments of Anatomy and Cell Biology, University of Alberta, Edmonton, AB, T6G 2S2, Canada, [c]Lipid and Lipoprotein Research Group and Department of Biochemistry, University of Alberta, Edmonton, AB, T6G 2S2, Canada

Introduction

Axonal growth of neurons is a process unlike any occurring in other types of cells, because the majority of the biosynthetic machinery of the cell (i.e., nucleus, ribosomes) is localized to the cell body, whereas the growth cone of the axon is often situated a large distance from the cell body. This unusual topology poses unique problems for the biogenesis and transport of membrane materials required for axonal growth. Until recently the dogma was that all membrane proteins and lipids required for axonal growth were synthesized in cell bodies and transported *via* anterograde transport into the axons (1–3). Indeed, ribosomes, the sites of protein synthesis, have been identified in cell bodies and possibly in dendrites (4), but not in axons. Similarly, the lipid components of axonal membranes were assumed to be synthesized in the cell bodies (1,2) and anterogradely transported into axons. Nevertheless, the source of axonal lipids had not been rigorously investigated in pure, intact, mammalian neurons. Some experiments—for example, in mouse sciatic nerves (5–8), extruded squid axoplasm (9,10) and rat brain synaptosomes (11)—had suggested that axons themselves might have the capacity to synthesize at least some of their own phospholipids. We have recently investigated the ability of axons of rat sympathetic neurons to synthesize lipids such as cholesterol, phospholipids and sphingolipids, and have examined which of these processes are essential for normal axonal elongation. In addition, we have studied whether or not alternative sources of these lipids can be used for axonal growth.

Unique Culture System for Studying Lipid Metabolism in Axons

For our studies we have cultured pure rat sympathetic neurons, derived from the superior cervical ganglia of one-day-old rats, in compartmented culture dishes (12). As illustrated in Fig. 8.1, neurons are plated in the center compartment of culture dishes that have been divided into three compartments. Growing axons extend at the rate of ~1 mm per day and enter the left and right compartments under the Teflon™ barriers and along the collagen tracks between the scratches. Each compartment

Compartmented culture

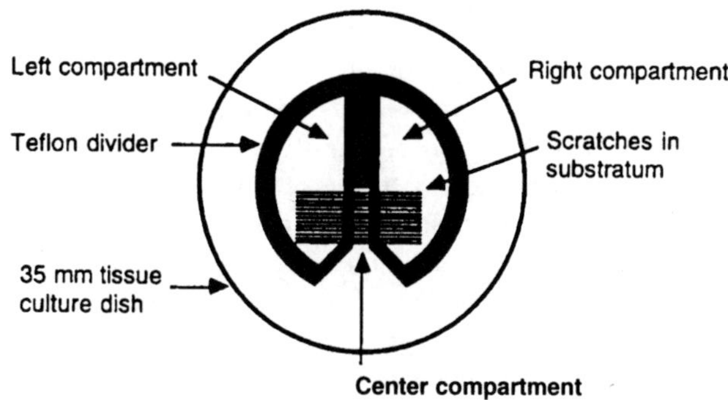

Enlargement of a single track

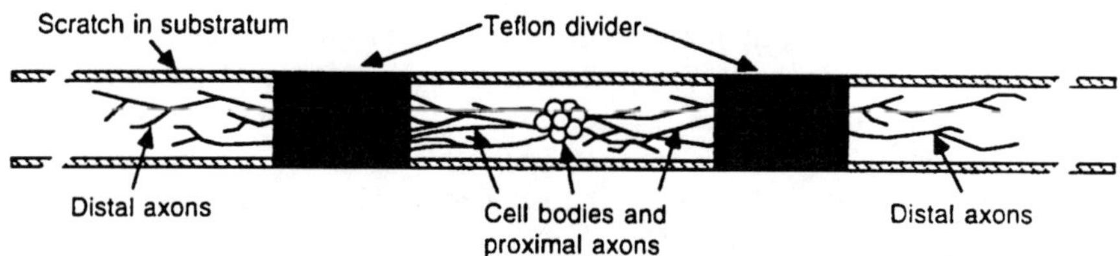

Fig. 8.1. Compartmented culture system for rat sympathetic neurons.

contains a separate fluid environment. The extension of the axons can be accurately measured under a microscope. The center compartment contains cell bodies and some proximal axons, whereas the left and right compartments contain pure distal axons without cell bodies.

This culture system has several major advantages compared to other models used for studying axonal growth (13,14). First, primary cultures of mammalian neurons, rather than transformed cell lines or nonmammalian neurons, can be studied. Second, the neurons are virtually free from contamination by other cell types, because cytosine arabinoside (which kills dividing cells) is added for the first few days of culture. Third, metabolic events occurring in distal axons can be studied independently of those occurring in cell bodies, because there is virtually no bulk flow of small molecules between compartments (12). Fourth, extension of the axons can be measured precisely. Another advantage of this culture system is that axons in the left compartment, for example, can be treated with a test reagent while axons in the right compartment are treated in a different way and so serve as internal controls.

Phospholipids Are Synthesized in Axons

The compartmented culture of sympathetic neurons provided an ideal system in which to investigate whether or not axons were capable of the synthesis of phospholipid components required for axonal growth. [*Methyl*-^{3}H]choline, a radiolabeled precursor of both phosphatidylcholine (PtdCho) and sphingomyelin, was added to either the center compartment (containing cell bodies with proximal axons) or to the left and right compartments (containing distal axons alone). Lipids were isolated from cellular material in each compartment and separated by thin-layer chromatography, and radioactivity was measured in PtdCho and sphingomyelin. When [^{3}H]choline was added to the center compartment, radiolabeled PtdCho and sphingomyelin were produced in that compartment, with small amounts of each being transported into distal axons (less than 5% of the amounts in cell bodies after 16 h) (15). On the other hand, when [^{3}H]choline was added to the axon-containing compartments alone, radioactive PtdCho and sphingomyelin were generated in the axons, suggesting that PtdCho and sphingomyelin synthesis occurred in axons (15). Analysis of the [^{3}H]choline-labeled precursors of PtdCho (i.e., choline, phosphocholine, and CDP-choline) in the three compartments revealed a lack of equilibration of these intermediates among the compartments (15). This observation suggests that the labeling of PtdCho and sphingomyelin in the axons was *not* the result of biosynthesis of the lipid within the cell bodies from radiolabeled precursors transported from distal axons, followed by anterograde movement of the lipid products from cell bodies to axons. Rather, the data imply that PtdCho and sphingomyelin are synthesized in axons.

As additional evidence that PtdCho is synthesized in axons, cell bodies and proximal axons were removed from the culture dish by vigorous washing, and the severed distal axons remaining in the side compartments were incubated with [*methyl*-^{3}H]choline for 5 h. The incorporation of radioactivity into PtdCho was the same as in axons of intact neurons (16). Thus, the attachment of cell bodies to the distal axons was not required for distal axons to convert [^{3}H]choline to PtdCho.

That axons have the capacity to synthesize PtdCho was also confirmed by measurement of the axonal activities of three enzymes involved in the CDP-choline pathway for PtdCho biosynthesis. choline kinase, CTP:phosphocholine cytidylyltransferase, and CDP-choline:diacylglycerol cholinephosphotransferase. The specific activities of these enzymes were of similar magnitude in cellular material isolated from the cell body–containing compartment, from distal axons, and from cultured rat hepatocytes (17). Because many enzymes involved in lipid synthesis are membrane-associated proteins of the endoplasmic reticulum (18), our observations also support the idea that endoplasmic reticulum membranes, or similar membranous structures, exist in axons (19,20).

PtdCho and sphingomyelin are not the only lipids synthesized in axons. Using similar radiolabeling experiments we demonstrated that phosphatidylethanolamine was synthesized in axons, both from the CDP-ethanolamine pathway and from decarboxylation of phosphatidylserine. In addition, phosphatidylserine, phosphatidylinositol, and fatty acids were shown to be made in axons (17).

Axonal Synthesis of PtdCho Is Required for Normal Axonal Growth

Although the radiolabeling experiments summarized above demonstrated that PtdCho was synthesized in axons, our experiments did not indicate what fraction of the PtdCho of distal axons was made locally in axons and what fraction was made in cell bodies and imported into axons. We, therefore, performed a double-labeling experiment in which [*methyl*-^{3}H]choline was added to the compartments containing cell bodies and [*methyl*-^{14}C]choline was added to the compartments containing distal axons. The specific radioactivities of choline in the media added to all three compartments were equalized. The amounts of [^{3}H]choline and [^{14}C]choline incorporated into axonal PtdCho were approximately equal, indicating that approximately half of the axonal PtdCho had been derived from [^{3}H]choline by synthesis in cell bodies, whereas half had been derived from [^{14}C]choline by local synthesis of PtdCho in distal axons (16). Since the central compartment, the source of [^{3}H]choline, contained proximal axons as well as cell bodies, we conclude that at least 50% of axonal PtdCho is synthesized *in situ* in axons.

Having shown that substantial amounts of axonal PtdCho were made in axons, we wished to determine whether or not PtdCho synthesis in axons was essential for axonal extension. Using the compartmented culture system for growth of sympathetic neurons, we inhibited PtdCho synthesis in axons by two approaches. First, choline, an obligatory precursor of PtdCho, was omitted from the culture medium. This treatment is a highly specific method by which to inhibit PtdCho biosynthesis (21). In compartmented cultures of neurons depleted of choline, the incorporation of [^{3}H]palmitate into PtdCho was inhibited by over 50%, indicating that PtdCho synthesis was inhibited by lack of choline (16). The neurons were then incubated under the following conditions:

- Choline depletion (CD) in the compartment containing cell bodies (CB), choline present in the distal axon–containing compartments
- CD in the distal axon–containing compartments (Ax), choline present in the cell body–containing compartment
- Choline depletion in all compartments (CD in CB + Ax)
- Choline present in all compartments (control)

As shown in Fig. 8.2, depletion of choline from the medium bathing the cell bodies did not affect the rate of axonal extension. However, when choline was omitted from either the medium bathing the distal axons or from the medium added to all compartments, axonal growth was severely compromised. The impact of choline deficiency on axonal extension became increasingly more severe as the duration of choline defi-

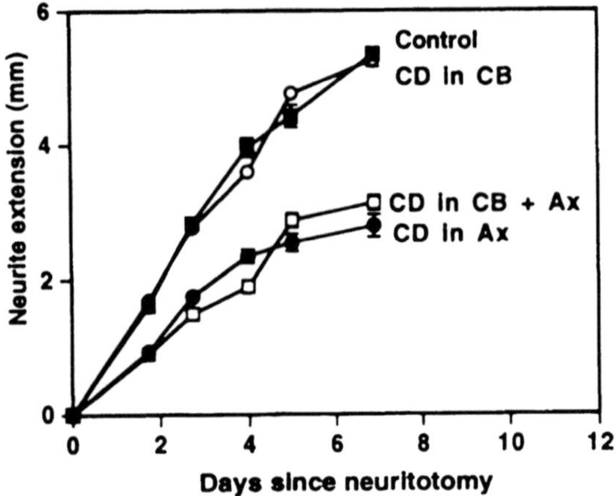

Fig. 8.2. Inhibition of neurite growth by choline deficiency (CD) in distal axons. Neurite extension was measured at the indicated times. Data are averages ± SEM from measurement of 62–64 tracks. The experiment was repeated three times with similar results. (*Source:* Posse de Chaves, E. *et al.* (1995) *J. Cell. Biol.* *128*, 913–918. Reprinted with permission.)

ciency was increased. In addition, the inhibitory effect of choline deficiency on neurite growth was reversed upon addition of choline to the culture medium of neurons that had been deprived of choline for 3 days (16).

In a parallel series of experiments, PtdCho biosynthesis was inhibited by addition of one of three alkylphosphocholines (dodecylphosphocholine, hexadecylphosphocholine, or octadecylphosphocholine) to the culture medium of compartmented neuron cultures. These compounds are antineoplastic agents that have been reported to inhibit PtdCho biosynthesis in Madin-Darby canine kidney cells (22,23). Our experiments showed that these three alkylphosphocholines inhibited PtdCho biosynthesis in sympathetic neurons by 36–60% (24) and impaired axonal elongation to an equivalent extent when added to distal axons, but not when added to cell bodies.

The experiments in which PtdCho biosynthesis was inhibited by choline deprivation or by the presence of alkylphosphocholines yielded the unexpected conclusion that axonal synthesis of PtdCho is necessary and sufficient for axonal extension. In contrast, synthesis of PtdCho in cell bodies is not required for axonal growth.

Cholesterol Synthesis in Cell Bodies Is Required for Axonal Growth of Cultured Neurons

Cholesterol is another major membrane lipid in all cell types, including neurons. Since we had observed that PtdCho, the major membrane phospholipid, was synthesized in axons, we next investigated the axonal synthesis of cholesterol by incubation of compartmented cultures of neurons with [^{14}C]acetate. Although active incorporation of the radiolabel into cholesterol occurred in the cell body–containing compartment, no synthesis of cholesterol was detected in distal axons (17). However, cholesterol synthesized in the cell body–containing compartment was efficiently transported into distal axons. Three days after the addition of [^{14}C]acetate to the cell body–containing compartment, radiolabeled cholesterol was completely equilibrated throughout the neuronal material in all three compartments (25). These observations indicated that cholesterol required for axonal growth could be supplied by anterograde transport from cell bodies and was sufficient for sustaining normal neurite extension in this culture system.

Cholesterol biosynthesis is known to be inhibited in several cell types by compounds such as pravastatin, which inhibit the rate-limiting enzyme of cholesterol biosynthesis: 3-hydroxy-3-methylglutaryl-CoA reductase (26). We have demonstrated that in rat sympathetic neurons pravastatin inhibited the incorporation of [1-^{14}C]acetate into cholesterol by 83% after 24 h (25). The compartmented neuron cultures were then incubated with pravastatin in either the cell body–containing compartment or the distal axon–containing compartments, and neurite extension was measured. In cultures that had been given pravastatin in the cell body–containing compartment, axonal extension was 45–55% less than in cultures grown in medium lacking pravastatin. As expected, since cholesterol synthesis was not detected in axons (17), addition of pravastatin to the distal axon–containing compartments did not affect axon growth (25). The inhibitory effect of pravastatin on axonal extension was specifically related to inhibition of 3-hydroxy-3-methylglutaryl-CoA reductase, because when the medium added to the cell body–containing compartment was supplemented with mevalonic acid (the product of the reaction catalyzed by the reductase), the inhibitory effect of pravastatin on neurite growth was reversed (25).

From these studies we conclude that cholesterol synthesis is required for axonal elongation. Moreover, the data suggest that cholesterol synthesis in cell bodies is sufficient to sustain normal axonal growth.

Cholesterol Can Be Supplied to Axons through Exogenous Delivery of Cholesterol or Lipoproteins

An alternative source of cholesterol for growing axons *in vivo* has been proposed to be lipoproteins such as those containing apolipoprotein E, or "recycled" cholesterol derived from degradation of myelin (27). We therefore investigated the ability of neurons to utilize exogenously delivered cholesterol for axon growth. Sympathetic neurons were plated in the three-compartment dishes, and axons were allowed to grow under the following conditions:

- With pravastatin in the cell body–containing compartment
- With pravastatin and cholesterol (incorporated into β-cyclodextrin) in the cell body–containing compartment

- With pravastatin in the cell body–containing compartment and cholesterol in the distal axon–containing compartments

- Without cholesterol and pravastatin in all three compartments.

In cultures that were given pravastatin in the cell body–containing compartment, axonal extension was impaired. However, in cultures given both pravastatin in the cell body–containing compartment and exogenous cholesterol (in either the cell body compartment or the distal axon–containing compartments), neurite growth was normal (25). These results indicate that axons of rat sympathetic neurons can use cholesterol exogenously supplied to either cell bodies or axons for biogenesis of axonal membranes.

In the circulation, one function of serum lipoproteins is to deliver cholesterol and other lipids to tissues. The presence of lipoproteins, particularly those containing apolipoproteins E or AI, has been observed in the vicinity of regenerating nerves (28). We therefore investigated the ability of serum lipoproteins to supply cholesterol to neurons for axonal growth. Three different classes of lipoproteins were used:

- Low-density lipoprotein (LDL), which contains apolipoprotein B but not apolipoprotein E

- High-density lipoprotein–2 (HDL-2), which contains apolipoproteins E, AI, and AII

- HDL-3, which contains apolipoproteins AI and AII but not apolipoprotein E

These lipoproteins were added to the different compartments of the cultured rat sympathetic neurons in which cholesterol biosynthesis had been inhibited by treatment of the cell bodies with pravastatin. The concentration of lipoproteins added was adjusted so that the same amount of total cholesterol was given in each case. When the lipoproteins were added to distal axons alone, all of the lipoproteins were able to overcome the inhibitory effect of pravastatin on axonal growth. However, when lipoproteins were added to the cell body–containing compartment, only LDL was as effective as cholesterol in restoring neurite growth; normal axonal extension did not resume when HDL-2 or HDL-3 was added to the cell body compartment of pravastatin-treated neurons (25). We speculate that the difference in the ability of the different classes of lipoproteins to rescue axonal growth when added to the cell bodies versus distal axons is related to different mechanisms of uptake of the lipoproteins.

These studies demonstrate that cholesterol can be supplied to growing axons from either endogenous synthesis or from exogenous delivery of cholesterol or lipoproteins. However, since HDL-3 contains no apolipoprotein E, and LDL contains no apolipoproteins E or AI, we conclude that neither of these apolipoproteins is required for delivery of lipoprotein cholesterol to distal axons. This conclusion is in agreement with studies in mice in which the genes for both apolipoproteins E and AI were disrupted but no neurological abnormalities were detected (29,30).

Lipoprotein Phosphatidylcholine Does Not Rescue Impaired Neurite Growth Caused by Choline Deficiency

As discussed above, when endogenous PtdCho biosynthesis in axons is inhibited, axonal growth is impaired (16). Since exogenously added lipoprotein cholesterol is able to overcome the disruption in axon growth caused by inhibition of endogenous cholesterol synthesis, we investigated whether or not PtdCho supplied by exogenously added lipoproteins could rescue the defect in axon growth caused by axonal choline deficiency. Sympathetic neurons were grown in compartmented culture dishes in the absence of choline in the distal axon–containing compartments. When choline was added to the distal axon–containing compartments, the normal rate of neurite growth resumed. However, when the lipoproteins LDL, HDL-2, or HDL-3 were added to the choline-deficient axons, neurite growth did not resume. In these experiments the concentration of cholesterol added in the form of lipoproteins was sufficient to restore normal axonal growth in neurons in which cholesterol synthesis had been inhibited. Moreover, the amount of choline delivered from PtdCho in the lipoproteins was 10 to 150 times higher than the choline content of normal culture medium (25).

Our conclusion from these experiments is that lipoproteins are unable to provide PtdCho, or precursors of PtdCho biosynthesis, for membrane biogenesis in distal axons.

Elevation of Ceramide Within Distal Neurites Inhibits Neurite Growth

Glycosphingolipids, which are major components of all eukaryotic cell membranes, are highly enriched in membranes of neurons. Several studies have suggested that sphingolipid synthesis is essential for normal growth of axons and dendrites (31–33). We investigated the role of sphingolipids in axonal growth by treatment of rat sympathetic neurons with two inhibitors of endogenous glycosphingolipid synthesis. The two inhibitors used were D,L-1-pheryl-2-palmitoylamino-3-morpholino-1-propanol (PPMP), which inhibits the synthesis of glucosylceramide from ceramide (34,35) (Fig. 8.3), and fumonisin B_1, which inhibits sphinganine *N*-acyltransferase and consequently inhibits the synthesis of dihydroceramide (36) (Fig. 8.3). Both fumonisin B_1 and PPMP potently inhibited glycosphingolipid synthesis in rat sympathetic neurons. Moreover, when PPMP was given to distal axons alone, neurite extension was 61% less than in cells incubated without PPMP. In contrast, when this inhibitor was added to the cell body–containing compartment, neurite growth was unaffected, even though glycosphingolipid synthesis was severely impaired. In addition, fumonisin B_1 did not inhibit axon growth when added to either cell bodies or axons, although sphingolipid biosynthesis was potently inhibited (37). Since both reagents inhibited sphingolipid synthesis, but only PPMP impaired

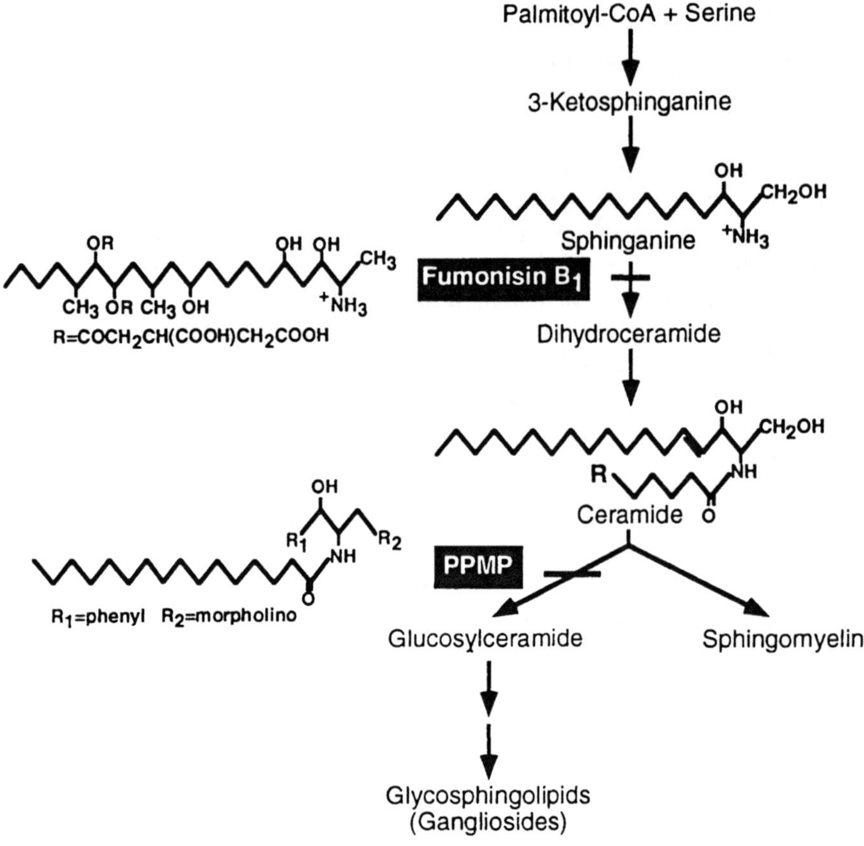

Fig. 8.3. Biosynthetic pathways for glycosphingolipids and sites of action of fumonisin B₁ and PPMP.

axonal growth whereas fumonisin B_1 did not, we conclude that PPMP is acting on neurite growth *via* a mechanism other than inhibition of sphingolipid synthesis.

One possible mode of action of these inhibitors on neurite growth is regulation of the levels of ceramide within the neurons. Ceramide has been identified as an important lipid second messenger and is reported to be involved in regulating cellular processes such as cell division and apoptosis (38,39). Since the two inhibitors act at different sites in the glycosphingolipid biosynthetic pathway (Fig. 8.3), we would anticipate that fumonisin might decrease, whereas PPMP might increase, ceramide levels. We therefore investigated the effects of PPMP and fumonisin B_1 on the incorporation of [^{3}H]palmitate into ceramide in rat sympathetic neurons. PPMP increased the incorporation of radioactivity into ceramide by ~2.5-fold, whereas in the presence of fumonisin B_1 the amount of radioactive ceramide was decreased by ~50% (37). Our results suggested, therefore, that elevated ceramide levels within the axons might be responsible for the inhibitory effect of PPMP on axon growth. This hypothesis was tested further by examination of the effects of the cell-permeable ceramide, C_6-ceramide, on neurite growth. Neurons treated in the cell body–containing compartment with C_6-ceramide elongated at the same rate as did untreated neurons. In contrast, when C_6-ceramide was added to distal axons, axon elongation was inhibited by 60%. Although we cannot rule out the possibility that the inhibition of axonal growth was due to a metabolite of ceramide rather than to ceramide itself, experiments using a fluorescent analog of C_6-ceramide showed that during the time frame of the experiments, 90% of the fluoresecent label remained in ceramide and only 2% was metabolized to ceramide-1-phosphate (37). One interesting implication from these experiments is that ceramide inhibits neurite growth only when its level is increased in distal axons, not when its level is increased in cell bodies. These results agree with the location of the observed effects of PPMP on neurite growth. We conclude, therefore, that when the concentration of the lipid second messenger ceramide is increased locally in distal axons, axonal growth is inhibited.

Conclusions

The experiments described above illustrate the importance of lipid metabolism in rat sympathetic neurons for regulation of axonal growth. We have shown that axonal extension requires the endogenous synthesis of PtdCho in distal axons. This requirement cannot be substituted by PtdCho synthesis in cell bodies or by supplying of exogenous PtdCho in the form of lipoproteins. In contrast, cholesterol synthesis is restricted to cell bodies, and cholesterol synthesized at this site is required for axonal growth in the absence of an exogenous supply. Alternatively, cholesterol can be supplied to neurons for axonal growth from an exogenous source, such as lipoproteins. Our studies also indicate that neurite growth is regulated by the level of ceramide within the axons and that an increase in axonal ceramide inhibits axonal extension.

References

1. Alberts, B., Bray, D., Lewis, J., Roberts, K., and Watson, J.D. (1989) *Molecular Biology of the Cell,* 2nd edn., pp. 1059–1136, Garland Press, New York.
2. Ledeen, R.W., and Eichberg, J. (1985) in *Phospholipids in Nervous Tissues,* Horrocks, L.A., Kanfer, J.N., and Porcellati, G., eds., Raven Press, Wiley, New York, pp. 135–172.
3. Toews, A.D., and Morrell, P. (1985) in *Phospholipids in the Nervous System,* Horrocks, L.A., Kanfer, J.N., and Porcellati, G., eds., Raven Press, New York, pp. 299–314.
4. Torre, E.R., and Steward, O. (1992) Demonstration of Local Protein Synthesis within Dendrites Using a New Cell Culture System That Permits the Isolation of Living Axons and Dendrites from Their Cell Bodies, *J. Neurosci. 12,* 762–772.
5. Gould, R.M. (1976) Inositol Lipid Synthesis Localized in Axons and Unmyelinated Fibers of Peripheral Nerve, *Brain Res. 117,* 169–174.
6. Gould, R.M., Holshek, J., Silverman, W., and Spivak, W.D. (1983) Localization of Phospholipid Synthesis to Schwann Cells and Axons, *J. Neurochem. 40,* 1300–1306.

7. Kumari-Siri, M.H., and Gould, R.M. (1980) Enzymes of Phospholipid Synthesis: Axonal vs. Schwann Cell Distribution, *Brain Res. 186*, 315–330.

8. Padilla, S., and Pope, C.N. (1991) Retrograde Axonal Transport of Locally Synthesized Phosphoinositides in the Rat Sciatic Nerve, *J. Neurochem. 56*, 415–422.

9. Gould, R.M., Spivak, W.D., Robertson, D., and Poznansky, M.J. (1983) Phospholipid Synthesis in the Squid Giant Axon: Enzymes of Phosphatidylinositol Metabolism, *J. Neurochem. 40*, 1300–1306.

10. Tanaka, T., Yamaguchi, H., Kishimoto, Y., and Gould, R.M. (1987) Lipid Metabolism in Various Regions of Squid Giant Nerve Fiber, *Biochim. Biophys. Acta 922*, 85–94.

11. Strosznajder, J., Radominska-Pyrek, A., and Horrocks, L.A. (1979) Choline and Ethanolamine Glycerolipid Synthesis in Isolated Synaptosomes of Rat Brain, *Biochim. Biophys. Acta 574*, 48–56.

12. Campenot, R.B. (1979) Independent Control of the Local Environment of Somas and Neurites, *Meths. Enzymol. 28*, 302–307.

13. Handelmann, G.E., Boyles, J.K., Weisgraber, K.H., Mahley, R.W., and Pitas, R.E. (1992) Effects of Apolipoprotein E, β-Very Low Density Lipoproteins, and Cholesterol on the Extension of Neurites by Rabbit Dorsal Root Ganglion Neurons *In Vitro, J. Lipid Res. 33*, 1677–1688.

14. Nathan, B.P., Bellosta, S., Sanan, D.A., Weisgraber, K.H., Mahley, R.W., and Pitas, R.E. (1994) Differential Effects of Apolipoproteins E3 and E4 on Neuronal Growth *In Vitro, Science 264*, 850–852.

15. Vance, J.E., Pan, D., Vance, D.E., and Campenot, R.B. (1991) Biosynthesis of Membrane Lipids in Rat Axons, *J. Cell Biol. 115*, 1061–1068.

16. Posse de Chaves, E., Vance, D.E., Campenot, R.B., and Vance, J.E. (1995) Axonal Synthesis of Phosphatidylcholine Is Required for Normal Axonal Growth in Rat Sympathetic Neurons, *J. Cell Biol. 128*, 913–918.

17. Vance, J.E., Pan, D., Campenot, R.B., Bussiere, M., and Vance, D.E. (1994) Evidence that the Major Membrane Lipids, Except Cholesterol, Are Made in Axons of Cultured Rat Sympathetic Neurons, *J. Neurochem. 62*, 329–337.

18. Vance, J.E., and Vance, D.E. (1988) Does Rat Liver Golgi Have the Capacity to Synthesize Phospholipids for Lipoprotein Secretion? *J. Biol. Chem. 263*, 5898–5909.

19. Rambourg, A., and Droz, B. (1989) Smooth Endoplasmic Reticulum and Axonal Transport, *J. Neurochem. 35*, 16–25.

20. Krijnse-Locker, J., Parton, R.G., Fuller, S.D., Griffiths, G., and Dotti, C.G. (1995) The Organization of the Endoplasmic Reticulum and Intermediate Compartment in Cultured Rat Hippocampal Neurons, *Molec. Biol. Cell 6*, 1315–1332.

21. Yao, Z., and Vance, D.E. (1988) The Active Synthesis of Phosphatidylcholine Is Required for Very Low Density Lipoprotein Secretion from Rat Hepatocytes, *J. Biol. Chem. 263*, 2998–3004.

22. Haase, R., Wieder, R., Geilen, C.C., and Reutter, W. (1991) The Phospholipid Analogue Hexadecylphosphocholine Inhibits Phosphatidylcholine Biosynthesis in Madin-Darby Canine Kidney Cells, *FEBS Lett. 288*, 129–132.

23. Wieder, T., Haase, A., Geilen, C.C., and Orfanos, C.E. (1995) The Effect of Two Synthetic Phospholipids on Cell Proliferation and Phosphatidylcholine Biosynthesis in Madin-Darby Canine Kidney Cells, *Lipids 30*, 389–393.

24. Posse de Chaves, E., Vance, D.E., Campenot, R.B., and Vance, J.E. (1995) Alkylphos-

phocholines Inhibit Choline Uptake and Phosphatidylcholine Biosynthesis in Rat Sympathetic Neurons and Impair Axonal Extension, *Biochem. J. 312*, 411–417.

25. Posse de Chaves, E.I., Rusiñol, A.E., Vance, D.E., Campenot, R.B., and Vance, J.E. (1997) Role of Lipoproteins in the Delivery of Lipids to Axons During Axonal Regeneration, *J. Biol. Chem. 272*, 30766–30773.

26. Tsujita, Y., Kuroda, M., Shimada, Y., Tanzawa, K., Arai, M., Kaneko, I., Tanaka, M., Masuda, H., Tarumi, C., Watanabe, Y., and Fujii, S. (1986) CS-514, a Competitive Inhibitor of 3-hydroxy-3-methylglutaryl Coenzyme A Reductase: Tissue-Selective Inhibition of Sterol Synthesis and Hypolipidemic Effect on Various Animal Species, *Biochim. Biophys. Acta 877*, 50–60.

27. Mahley, R.W. (1988) Apolipoprotein E: Cholesterol Transport Protein with Expanding Role in Cell Biology, *Science 240*, 622–630.

28. Boyles, J.K., Zoellner, C.D., Anderson, L.J., Kosik, L.M., Pitas, R.E., Weisgraber, K.H., Hui, D.Y., Mahley, R.W., Gebicke-Haerter, P.J., Ignatius, M.J., and Shooter, E.M. (1989) A Role for Apolipoprotein E, Apolipoprotein A-1, and Low Density Lipoprotein Receptors in Cholesterol Transport During Regeneration and Remyelination of the Rat Sciatic Nerve, *J. Clin. Invest. 83*, 1015–1031.

29. Popko, B., Goodrum, J.F., Bouldin, T.W., Zhang, S.H., and Maeda, N. (1993) Nerve Regeneration Occurs in the Absence of Apolipoprotein E in Mice, *J. Neurochem. 60*, 1155–1158.

30. Goodrum, J.F., Bouldin, T.W., Zhang, S.H., Maeda, N., and Popko, B. (1995) Nerve Regeneration and Cholesterol Reutilization Occur in the Absence of Apolipoproteins E and A1 in Mice, *J. Neurochem. 64*, 408–416.

31. Harel, R., and Futerman, A.H. (1993) Inhibition of Sphingolipid Synthesis Affects Axonal Outgrowth in Cultured Hippocampal Neurons, *J. Biol. Chem. 19*, 14476–14481.

32. Schwartz, A., Rapaport, E., Hirschberg, K., and Futerman, A.H. (1995) A Regulatory Role for Sphingolipids in Neuronal Growth, *J. Biol. Chem. 270*, 10990–10998.

33. Furuya, S., Ono, E., and Hirabayashi, Y. (1995) Sphingolipid Biosynthesis Is Necessary for Dendrite Growth and Survival of Cerebellar Purkinje Cells in Culture, *J. Neurochem. 65*, 1551–1561.

34. Inokuchi, J., and Radin, N.S. (1987) Preparation of the Active Isomer of 1-phenyl-2-decanoylamino-3-morpholino-1-propanol, Inhibitor of Murine Glucocerebroside Synthetase, *J. Lipid Res. 28*, 565–471.

35. Abe, A., Inokuchi, J., Jimbo, M., Shimeno, H., Nagamatsu, A., Shayman, G.S., and Radin, N.S. (1992) Improved Inhibitors of Glucosylceramide Synthase, *J. Biochem. 111*, 191–196.

36. Wang, E., Norred, W.P., Bacon, C.W., Riley, R.T., and Merrill, A.H. (1991) Inhibition of Sphingolipid Biosynthesis by Fumonisins, *J. Biol. Chem. 22*, 14486–14490.

37. Posse de Chaves, E.I., Bussière, M., Vance, D.E., Campenot, R.B., and Vance, J.E. (1997) Elevation of Ceramide within Distal Neurites Inhibits Neurite Growth in Cultured Rat Sympathetic Neurons, *J. Biol. Chem. 272*, 3028–3035.

Lowe Syndrome: A Human Inborn Error of Phosphatidylinositol Metabolism

Sharon F. Suchy and Robert L. Nussbaum

Genetic Disease Research Branch, National Human Genome Research Institute,
National Institutes of Health, Bethesda, MD

The Oculocerebrorenal Syndrome of Lowe

The oculocerebrorenal syndrome of Lowe (Lowe syndrome) is a rare, X-linked disorder which is characterized by bilateral congenital cataracts, renal tubular dysfunction, and neurological deficits including hypotonia, intellectual impairment, seizures, and behavioral abnormalities (1,2). The gene (OCRL1) that, when defective, causes Lowe syndrome was isolated by positional cloning (3).

OCRL1 Encodes a PtdIns(4,5)P$_2$ 5-Phosphatase

The predicted amino acid sequence of the OCRL1 gene product (ocrl1) provided the first clues as to its function. The ocrl1 protein has 53% amino acid identity and 71% similarity to an inositol polyphosphate 5-phosphatase, INPP5Bp (3). This enzyme catalyzes the hydrolysis of the 5-position phosphate from the inositol ring of soluble inositol 1,4,5-triphosphate [Ins(1,4,5)P$_3$]. The strong sequence homology between ocrl1 and INPP5Bp indicated that ocrl1 might have Ins(1,4,5)P$_3$ 5-phosphatase activity. However, we found no evidence that this activity was deficient in fibroblasts or lymphocytes from patients with Lowe syndrome. This led us to investigate another 5-phosphatase of the phosphatidylinositol pathway that catalyzes a very similar reaction: phosphatidylinositol 4,5-bisphosphate [PtdIns(4,5)P$_2$] 5-phosphatase. PtdIns(4,5)P$_2$ 5-phosphatase catalyzes the hydrolysis of a phosphate from the 5 position of the inositol ring from membrane-bound PtdIns(4,5)P$_2$. Lowe-patient fibroblasts were found to be deficient in PtdIns(4,5)P$_2$ 5-phosphatase activity (4).

Immunoprecipitation and overexpression experiments were performed to determine that ocrl1 was directly responsible for the PtdIns(4,5)P$_2$ 5-phosphatase activity. For these studies we used purified polyclonal antibodies to ocrl1 (5), made to the N-terminus of the ocrl1 protein—a region with little homology to INPP5Bp. In immunoprecipitation experiments, most of the protein was precipitated from fibroblast cell lysates (as demonstrated by western analysis) along with most of the PtdIns(4,5)P$_2$ 5-phosphatase activity (4). Transfection of OCRL1 into COS 7 cells resulted in a dramatic increase in ocrl1 expression along with an increase in PtdIns(4,5)P$_2$ 5-phosphatase activity, showing that ocrl1 was required for the

PtdIns(4,5)P$_2$ 5-phosphatase activity. These results were in agreement with a report by Zhang and colleagues, who found that a partial ocrl1 protein, overexpressed in baculovirus, had PtdIns(4,5)P$_2$ 5-phosphatase activity (6). Together these results demonstrated that ocrl1 was a PtdIns(4,5)P$_2$ 5-phosphatase.

This finding makes it possible to do direct biochemical testing to confirm the diagnosis of Lowe syndrome (7). OCRL1 is expressed in fibroblasts but not in lymphocytes. All Lowe-patient fibroblasts are markedly deficient in PtdIns(4,5)P$_2$ 5-phosphatase activity, with only about 7% of control activity on average (see Table 9.1). Most Lowe-patient fibroblasts have no detectable ocrl1 by western analysis, although several patients express some ocrl1 at markedly decreased levels. In several of the patients' fibroblasts that express protein, the mutations in ocrl1 were found to be point mutations in one of the highly conserved regions of ocrl1 (8,9). A patient fibroblast line with one of the lowest PtdIns(4,5)P$_2$ 5-phosphatase activities of 23 patients studied had approximately 50% of the control amount of ocrl1, as determined by western analysis. In this cell line a point mutation was found in one of six highly conserved motifs of ocrl1, shared by a number of PtdIns(4,5)P$_2$ 5-phosphatases and a protein with Ins(1,4,5)P$_3$ 5-phosphatase activity (Fig. 9.1). This makes it likely that this conserved motif is part of an inositol 5-phosphatase functional domain.

Roles for PtdIns(4,5)P$_2$

The substrate for PtdIns(4,5)P$_2$ 5-phosphatase, PtdIns(4,5)P$_2$, has several important functions in the cell (Fig. 9.2). PtdIns(4,5)P$_2$ has a well-established role in signal transduction in the generation of the second messengers Ins(1,4,5)P$_3$ and diacylglycerol *via* phospholipase C. PtdIns(4,5)P$_2$ is also the substrate for phosphatidylinositol 3-kinase, which forms the second messenger PtdIns(3,4,5)P$_3$ (10,11). In addition to the generation of second messengers, PtdIns(4,5)P$_2$ can bind to actin-binding proteins to promote actin polymerization (12,13). PtdIns(4,5)P$_2$ plays a role in the regulation of Golgi vesicular transport (14–16) and has also been shown to be involved in the activation of proteins that are involved in endocytic or synaptic vesicle transport (17). For example, PtdIns(4,5)P$_2$ activates dynamin, which has been proposed to play a role in synaptic vesicle recycling along with synaptojanin, a known PtdIns(4,5)P$_2$ 5-phosphatase (18).

TABLE 9.1

PtdIns(4,5)P$_2$ Phosphatase Activity in Human Fibroblasts

Fibroblasts	Activity (Mean ± SD) nmol/min/mg protein	Number tested
Unaffected	6.41 ± 0.81	7
Lowe	0.55 ± 0.29	23

OCRL1	S D H K P V S A L F H I
HumInpp5b	S D H K P V S S V F D I
Synaptojanin	S D H R P V V A L I D I
Hum51C	S D H S P V F G T F E V
SJL1	S D H R P V Y A I F R A
SJL2	S D H K P V Y A AY R A
SJL3	S D H R P V Y A AY R A
HumInpp5a	G D H K P V F L A F R I
PHL255*	S D R K P V S A L F H I

*Lowe-patient fibroblast line

Fig. 9.1. A highly conserved motif shared by a number of proteins with inositol phosphatase activity.

Subcellular Localization of ocrl1

Immunocytochemical studies performed in our laboratory have demonstrated that ocrl1 is predominantly a Golgi-localized protein (5). This information provides us with some important clues as to how ocrl1 functions in the cell. $PtdIns(4,5)P_2$ is an activator of two proteins known to be involved in Golgi trafficking: ADP ribosylation factor GTPase activating protein (ARF-GAP) and phospholipase D (PLD). $PtdIns(4,5)P_2$ has a stimulatory effect on ARF-GAP, resulting in the formation of ARF-GDP, the inactive form of ARF. The active form of ARF, ARF-GTP, is required for the binding of coat proteins to vesicles and their budding off from the membrane. ARF-GTP also activates PLD, converting phosphatidylcholine to choline and phosphatidic acid—the latter which potentiates the effect of $PtdIns(4,5)P_2$ on ARF-GAP.

How Might a Defective ocrl1 Protein Cause Lowe Syndrome?

Because of the Golgi localization of ocrl1, we speculate that the deficiency of this $PtdIns(4,5)P_2$ 5-phosphatase may impair Golgi vesicular transport. Deficient ocrl1 may result in elevated levels of $PtdIns(4,5)P_2$, which activates ARF-GAP to convert active ARF-GTP to inactive ARF-GDP, thus disrupting Golgi vesicular transport (Fig. 9.2). While a total disruption of Golgi transport would be expected to be lethal, a partial, protein-specific or tissue-specific disruption of Golgi transport may lead to

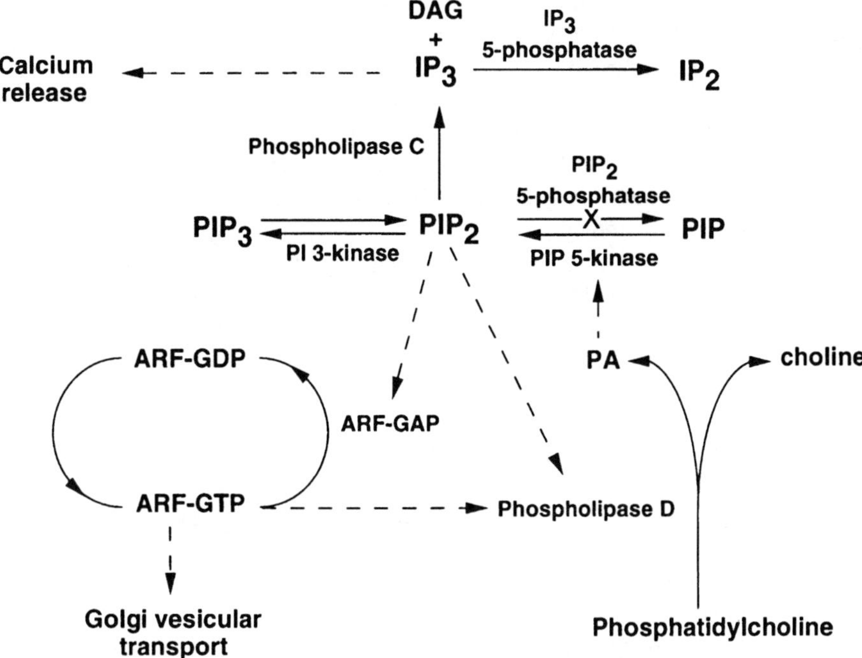

Fig. 9.2. The phosphatidylinositol pathway. *Abbreviations:* ARF GAP, ADP ribosylation factor GTPase activating protein (ARF-GAP); ARF-GDP, ADP ribosylation factor–guanosine diphosphate; ARF-GTP, ADP ribosylation factor–guanosine triphosphate; DAG, diacylglycerol; IP_2, inositol 1,4-diphosphate; IP_3, inositol 1,4,5-triphosphate [Ins(1,4,5)P_3]; PA, phosphatidic acid; PI, phosphatidylinositol; PIP, phosphatidylinositol 4-phosphate; PIP_2, phosphatidylinositol 4,5-bisphosphate [PtdIns(4,5)P_2]; PIP_3, phosphatidylinositol 3,4,5-triphosphate [PtdIns(3,4,5)P_3].

abnormal trafficking of proteins to the cell surface and affect interactions between cells or between cells and the substratum. Abnormal cell-surface properties might result in defective development or function of highly specialized tissues consistently affected in Lowe syndrome—for example, the lens or renal epithelia—to produce the cataracts and renal tubular dysfunction of Lowe syndrome.

A deficiency of PtdIns(4,5)P_2 phosphatose might be expected to produce elevated PtdIns(4,5)P_2 levels; however, no difference was found in whole-cell PtdIns(4,5)P_2 levels between Lowe and normal fibroblasts (Nussbaum, R.L., unpublished data). Recently, Zhang and colleagues reported a two-fold elevation in whole-cell PtdIns(4,5)P_2 levels between Lowe and normal kidney cell lines transformed using different viruses (19). Although one might ask whether a two-fold elevation in whole-cell PtdIns(4,5)P_2 would be sufficient to affect Golgi trafficking or other cell processes, this degree of elevation may reflect a substantial increase in PtdIns(4,5)P_2 levels in certain subcellular compartments. It is well established that distinct metabolic pools of PtdIns(4,5)P$_2$ are found in different subcellular compartments (20–22). These metabolic pools may result from physical compartmentalization by subcellular membranes or from interactions of PtdIns(4,5)P$_2$ with structural proteins such as actin-binding proteins (23). Therefore, alterations of PtdIns(4,5)P$_2$ levels in the Golgi apparatus, where ocrl1 is localized, may be quite different from that observed in the whole cell. It will be important to study Golgi PtdIns(4,5)P$_2$ levels in Lowe cells.

Nevertheless, the finding of elevated PtdIns (4,5)P$_2$ levels in kidney cells from Lowe patients but not in fibroblasts is interesting since the kidney is one of the tissues affected in Lowe syndrome. This may indicate that some cell types (such as fibroblasts) may be able to "correct" for abnormal subcellular levels of PtdIns(4,5)P$_2$. In fact, variations in the tissue and subcellular distributions of isozymes of other PtdIns(4,5)P$_2$-metabolizing enzymes (such as other PtdIns(4,5)P$_2$ 5-phosphatases, PtdIns(4)P 5-kinase, phospholipase C, and PtdIns(4,5)P$_2$ 3-kinase (24–27) suggest that PtdIns(4,5)P$_2$ is metabolized by tissue- or subcellular compartment-specific mechanisms.

Since PtdIns(4,5)P$_2$ has numerous cellular roles, Golgi trafficking may not be the only process affected in Lowe syndrome. In fact, there is an interesting relationship between vesicular transport, actin binding proteins and PtdIns(4,5)P$_2$ 5-phosphatase. A yeast mutant, SAC1, is able to correct both secretory defects and actin-binding defects (28,29). Moreover, synaptojanin, a synaptic-vesicle protein, contains both an actin-binding domain (shared homology with SAC1P) and a PtdIns(4,5)P$_2$ 5-phosphatase domain (17). Synaptojanin provides evidence of the importance of having a PtdIns(4,5)P$_2$ 5-phosphatase closely associated with actin. The phenotype in Lowe syndrome may be in part due to abnormal polymerization of the actin produced by abnormal local levels of PtdIns(4,5)P$_2$.

An OCRL1 Knockout Mouse

Because of the importance of studying metabolism in specific tissues that are most affected by the gene defect, our lab created a genetic knockout of OCRL1 in mice by homologous recombination (30). These mice, however, appeared phenotypically normal. Fibroblasts from these mouse knockouts had a higher residual PtdIns(4,5)P$_2$ 5-phosphatase activity than Lowe-patient fibroblasts (30). This suggests that in the mouse there is another PtdIns(4,5)P$_2$ 5-phosphatase that compensates for the ocrl1 activity. Alternatively, there might be some important developmental differences in the lens, kidney, or brain of mice that may make them less susceptible to the deficiency.

Summary

Lowe syndrome is the first known defect in phosphatidylinositol metabolism in higher eukaryotes. This disorder is due to a deficiency of a Golgi-localized

PtdIns(4,5)P$_2$ 5-phosphatase. A deficiency of this enzyme may disrupt Golgi vesicular transport and result in aberrant trafficking of proteins to the cell surface, abnormal cell–cell interactions, and developmental or functional abnormalities in particular tissues. In the kidney such abnormalities may disrupt the formation of tight junctions, which restrict the flow of metabolites between cells. In the lens such abnormalities may alter cell–cell junctions of fiber or epithelial cells that are important in normal lens development and function.

We are just beginning to understand how a defect in a Golgi-localized PtdIns(4,5)P$_2$ 5-phosphatase results in Lowe syndrome. We believe that the study of this disorder will provide critical clues about the important role of phospholipid metabolism in normal cell function.

References

1. Lowe, C.U., Terrey, M., and MacLachlan, E.A. (1952) Organic Aciduria, Decreased Renal Ammonia Production, Hydrophthalmos, and Mental Retardation: A Clinical Entity, *Am. J. Dis. Child. 83*, 164.
2. Charnas, L., and Nussbaum, R.L. (1995) in *The Metabolic Basis of Inherited Disease*, Scriver, C.R., Beaudet, A.L. Sly, W.S. and Valle, D., eds., McGraw-Hill, New York, vol. III, pp. 3705–3716.
3. Attree, O., Olivos, I.M., Okabe, I., Bailey, L.C., Nelson, D.L., Lewis, R.A., McInnes, R.R., and Nussbaum, R.L. (1992) The Lowe Oculocerebrorenal Syndrome Gene Encodes a Protein Highly Homologous to Inositol Polyphosphate-5-Phosphatase, *Nature 358*, 239–242.
4. Suchy, S.F., Olivos-Glander, I.M., and Nussbaum, R.L. (1995) Lowe Syndrome, a Deficiency of a Phosphatidylinositol 4,5-Bisphosphate 5-Phosphatase in the Golgi Apparatus, *Hum. Molec. Genet. 4*, 2245–2250.
5. Olivos-Glander, I.M., Jänne, P.A., and Nussbaum, R.L. (1995) The Oculocerebrorenal Syndrome Gene Product Is a 105 kDa Protein Localized to the Golgi Complex, *Am. J. Hum. Genet. 57*, 817–823.
6. Zhang, X., Jefferson, A.B., Auethavekiat, V., and Majerus, P.W. (1995) The Protein Deficient in Lowe Syndrome Is a Phosphatidylinositol-4,5-Bisphosphate 5-Phosphatase, *Proc. Natl. Acad. Sci. USA 92*, 4853–4856.
7. Suchy, S.F., Olivos-Glander, I.M., Horwitz, J.A., and Nussbaum, R.L. (1996) Prenatal Biochemical Testing for Lowe Syndrome, *Am. J. Hum. Genet. 59*, A330.
8. Leahey, A., Charnas, L.R., and Nussbaum, R.L. (1993) Nonsense Mutations in the *OCRL-1* Gene in Patients with the Oculocerebrorenal Syndrome of Lowe, *Hum. Molec. Genet. 2*, 461–463.
9. Lin, T., Suchy, S.F., Orrison, B.M., Leahey, A. Lewis, R.A., and Nussbaum, R.L. (1996) Mutations in the *OCRL1* Gene in the Oculocerebrorenal Syndrome, *Am. J. Hum. Genet. 59*, A269.
10. Varticovski, L., Harrison-Findik, D., Keeler, M.L. and Susa, M. (1994) Role of PI 3-Kinase in Mitogenesis, *Biochim. Biophys. Acta 1226*, 1–11.
11. Toker, A., Bachelot, C. Chen, C.-S., Falck, J.R., Hartwig, J.H., Cantley, L.C., and Kovacsovics, T.J. (1995) Phosphorylation of the Platelet p47 Phosphoprotein is Mediated by the Lipid Products of Phosphoinositide 3-Kinase, *J. Biol. Chem. 270*, 29525–29531.

12. Janmey, P.A. (1994) Phosphoinositides and Calcium as Regulators of Cellular Actin Assembly and Disassembly, *Annu. Rev. Physiol. 56*, 169–191.

13. Yu, F.-X., Sun, H.-Q., Janmey, P.A., and Yin, H.L. (1992) Identification of a Polyphosphoinositide-Binding Sequence in an Actin Monomer-Binding Domain of Gelsolin, *J. Biol. Chem. 267*, 14616–14621.

14. Randazzo, P.A., and Kahn, R.A. (1994) GTP Hydrolysis by ADP-Ribosylation Factor Is Dependent on Both an ADP-Ribosylation Factor GTPase-Activating Protein and Acid Phospholipids, *J. Biol. Chem. 269*, 10758–10763.

15. Pertile, P., Liscovitch, M., Chalifa, V., and Cantley, L.C. (1995) Phosphatidylinositol 4,5 Bisphosphate Synthesis Is Required for Activation of Phospholipase D in U937 Cells, *J. Biol. Chem. 270*, 5130–5135.

16. Terui, T., Kahn, R.A., and Randazzo, P.A. (1994) Effects of Acid Phospholipids on Nucleotide Exchange Properties of ADP)-Ribosylation Factor 1. Evidence for Specific Interaction with Phosphatidylinositol 4,5-Bisphosphate, *J. Biol. Chem. 269*, 28130–28135.

17. McPhearson, P.S., Garcia, E.P., Slepnev, V.I., David, C., Zhang, X., Grabs, D., Sossin, W.S., Bauerfeind, R., Nemoto, Y., and De Camilli, P. (1996) A Presynaptic Inositol-5-Phosphatase, *Nature 379*, 353–357.

18. Tuma, P.L., Stachniak, M.C., and Collins, C.A. (1993) Activation of Dynamin GTPase by Acidic Phospholipids and Endogenous Rat Brain Vesicles, *J. Biol. Chem. 268*, 17204–17206.

19. Zhang, X., Hartz, P., Philip, E., Racusen, L.C., and Majerus, P.W. (1998) Cell Lines from Kidney Proximal Tubules of a Patient with Lowe Syndrome Lack OCRL Inositol Polyphosphate 5-Phosphatase and Accumulate Phosphatidylinositol 4,5-Bisphosphate, *J. Biol. Chem. 273*, 1574–1582.

20. Koreh, K. and Monaco, M.E. (1986) The Relationship of Hormone-Sensitive and Hormone-Insensitive Phosphatidylinositol to Phosphatidylinositol 4,5-Bisphosphate in the WRK-1 Cell, *J. Biol. Chem. 261*, 88–91.

21. Vickers, J.D., and Mustard, J.F. (1986) The Phosphoinositides Exist in Multiple Metabolic Pools in Rabbit Platelets, *Biochem. J. 238*, 411–417.

22. King, C.E., Stephens, L.R., Hawkins, P.T., Guy, G.R., and Michell, R.H. (1987) Multiple Metabolic Pools of Phosphoinositides and Phosphatidate in Human Erythrocytes Incubated in a Medium That Permits Rapid Transmembrane Exchange of Phosphate, *Biochem. J. 244*, 209–217.

23. Goldschmidt-Clermont, P.J., Kim, J.W., Machesky, L.M., Rhee, S.G., and Pollard, T.D. (1991) Regulation of Phospholipase C-gamma 1 by Profilin and Tyrosine Phosphorylation, *Science 251*, 1231–1233.

24. Imai, A., Rebecchi, M.J., and Gershengorn, M.C. (1986) Differential Regulation by Phosphatidylinositol 4,5-Bisphosphate of Pituitary Plasma-Membrane and Cytosolic Phosphoinositol Kinase, *Biochem. J. 240*, 341–348.

25. Bazenet, C.E., Ruano, A.R., Brockman, J.L., and Anderson, R.A. (1990) The Human Erythrocyte Contains Two Forms of Phosphatidylinositol-4-Phosphate 5-Kinase Which Are Differentially Active Toward Membranes, *J. Biol. Chem. 265*, 18012–18022.

26. Brooksbank, C.E.L., Hutchings, A., Butcher, G.W., Irvine, R. F., and Divecha, N. (1993) Monoclonal Antibodies to Phosphatidylinositol 4-Phosphate 5-Kinase: Distribution and Intracellular Localization of the C Isoform, *Biochem. J. 291*, 77–82.

27. Hope, H.M., and Pike, L.J. (1994) Purification and Characterization of a Polyphosphoinositide Phosphatase from Rat Brain, *J. Biol. Chem. 269*, 23648–23654.

28. Cleves, A.E., Novick, P.J., and Bankaitis, V.A. (1989) Mutations in the SAC1 Gene Suppress Defects in Yeast Golgi and Yeast Actin Function, *J. Cell Biol. 109*, 2939–2950.
29. Novick, P., Osmond, B.C., and Botstein, D.D. (1989) Suppressors of Yeast Actin Mutations, *Genetics 121*, 659–674.
30. Jänne, P.A., Suchy, S.F., Bernard, D., McDonald, M., Crawley, J., Wynshaw-Boris, A., Westphal, H., and Nussbaum, R.L. (1998) Functional Overlap Between Murine *Inpp5b* and *ocrl1* May Explain Why Deficiency of the Murine Ortholog for OCRL1 Does Not Cause Lowe Syndrome in Mice, *J. Clin. Invest. 101*, 2042–2053.

Chapter 10

Alterations in Myocardial Phospholipid Metabolism During Myocardial Ischemia

Richard W. Gross

Division of Bioorganic Chemistry and Molecular Pharmacology, Washington University School of Medicine, St. Louis, MO 63110

Introduction

Myocardial ischemia is accompanied by multiple changes in sugar and lipid metabolism, including alterations in glycolytic flux, phospholipolysis, and fatty acid β-oxidation (1–4). As a result of these metabolic alterations, critical changes in energy production and utilization occur in cardiac myocytes during the ischemic process; these changes are accompanied by resultant alterations in myocardial hemodynamic properties, electrophysiologic function, and cellular integrity (5). In myocardium, as in other tissues, the function of transmembrane proteins is modulated by the chemical composition, physical properties, and molecular dynamics of their surrounding phospholipid constituents. During myocardial ischemia, a variety of factors contribute to accelerated phospholipolysis of the sarcolemmal membrane, resulting in the accumulation of biologically active lipid metabolites (e.g., arachidonic acid and lysophospholipids); these metabolites mediate many of the sequelae of myocardial ischemia through their effects on ion channel function, cellular membrane permeability, and receptor-effector coupling (6–9). Moreover, recent studies have now demonstrated the importance of the coupling between accelerated glycolysis and accelerated phospholipolysis during myocardial ischemia. The purpose of this chapter is to review the role of plasmalogens (highly specialized phospholipid constituents present in myocardial sarcolemmal membranes), to discuss the enzymes that mediate their catabolism, and to focus on recent insights into the biochemical mechanisms that mediate the regulation of myocardial phospholipase A_2 during the ischemic process.

Phospholipid Composition of Myocardial Sarcolemmal Membranes

Although it has been over 70 years since Feulgen's initial description of plasmalogens in biologic tissues (10), their functional role in cellular metabolism and homeostasis is just beginning to be elucidated. Plasmalogens are distinguished from conventional diacyl phospholipids by virtue of the presence of two sp^2-hybridized carbon atoms in the proximal portion of the *sn*-1 aliphatic chain. The presence of the vinyl ether linkage imparts specific constraints on the conformation and dynamics of plasmalogen molecular species, which differ dramatically from those of their diacyl phospholipid counterparts (11–15). In cardiac myocytes, the sarcolemmal membrane is responsible for the electrophysiologic properties of each cell, which reflect the cumulative influences of the kinetic characteristics of multiple ion channels, the intrinsic permeability properties of the sarcolemmal membrane bilayer, and the inter-action between complex arrays of heteromultimeric ion channels and their surrounding lipid constituents. In cardiac sarcolemma from many animal species (including humans), plasmalogens are the predominant phospholipid subclass present (16). Moreover, plasmalogen molecular species are highly enriched in arachidonic acid (17). For example, in canine myocardial sarcolemmal membranes 57% of choline glycerophospholipids and 64% of ethanolamine glycerophospho-lipids consisted of plasmalogen molecular species (16). Furthermore, 75% of sarcolemmal ethanolamine glycerophospholipids contained arachidonic acid esteri-fied to the *sn*-2 position (16). As will be seen from the following discussion, the marked enrichment of plasmalogen molecular species in the sarcolemmal membrane provides a unique environment for the function of highly specialized transmembrane proteins. Furthermore, the enrichment of arachidonic acid in plasmalogen molecular species serves as a specific pool for the liberation of biologically active eicosanoids by plasmalogen-selective phospholipases in myocardium. Through these conjoint actions—the provision of a specific chemical environment and a pool of latent biologically active lipids awaiting activation by enzymatic release—plasmalogens serve to fulfill specific functional roles in myocardial physiology, as will be shown.

Molecular Structure and Organizational Dynamics of Plasmalogen Molecular Species

The molecular dynamics of vesicles composed of plasmenylcholine and phos-phatidylcholine have been quantified utilizing electron spin resonance (ESR), deuterium magnetic resonance (^{2}H NMR), and fluorescence spectroscopy (11–15). ESR shows substantial differences in the order parameters for both 5-doxylstearate (5-DS) and 16-doxylstearate (16-DS) probes between vesicles composed of plas-menylcholine and those composed of phosphatidylcholine (e.g., $S = 0.592$ *vs.* 0.487 for 5-DS, and 0.107 *vs.* 0.099 for 16-DS, at 38°C.) (11). Furthermore, ^{2}H NMR spec-troscopy demonstrates that the order parameter of plasmenylcholine is greater than that of phosphatidylcholine for one of the two diastereotopic deuterons located at the C_2 carbon of the *sn*-2 fatty acyl chain (11). These results demonstrate that plas-menylcholine vesicles are more ordered than phosphatidylcholine vesicles, both in the interior of the membrane and at regions near the hydrophobic-hydrophilic inter-face. Experiments utilizing binary dispersions of cholesterol with each phospholipid subclass demonstrate that cholesterol results in substantial immobilization of phos-pholipids in both subclasses (18). Furthermore, although motion for both phospholipid subclasses is highly anisotropic, specific axes through which at least some types of motion occur for these phospholipid subclasses are separate and distinct. Taken together, these results demonstrate that membrane domains enriched in plasmalogen molecular species provide a unique molecular environment that differs markedly from that produced by diacyl phospholipids.

To identify further the specific chemical differences underlying the distinct molecular dynamics of plasmalogen and diacyl phospholipid subclasses, the conformation of plasmenylcholine near the hydrophobic–hydrophilic interface in membrane bilayers was studied through truncated driven nuclear Overhauser enhancement (12). Experiments demonstrated that the β-vinyl ether proton in plasmenylcholine was in close spatial proximity and nearly equidistant to both the α- and β-methylene protons of the sn-2 aliphatic chain (12). These results differ dramatically from those obtained for phosphatidylcholine bilayers, where the proximal portion of the sn-2 acyl chain is bent, coursing parallel to the plane of the membrane. These results demonstrate that modest alterations in covalent structure (i.e., the two sp^2 carbon atoms in the proximal portion of the sn-1 acyl chain) have substantial effects on molecular conformation of phospholipid bilayers.

Plasmalogens Mediate Phospholipid Subclass–Specific Alterations in Ion Transport Kinetics across Biologic Membranes

Although the predominance of plasmalogens in electrically active membranes is well known, identification of the molecular mechanisms through which the vinyl ether linkage facilitates electrophysiologic function has remained elusive. Recently, we demonstrated that the kinetics of both carrier-mediated (i.e., valinomycin) (19) and ion channel-mediated (gramicidin) (20) ion flux are substantially different in membranes composed of plasmalogen molecular species in comparison to their diacyl and alkyl ether choline glycerophospholipid counterparts. For example, the rank order of valinomycin-mediated K^+/Na^+ exchange was plasmenylcholine > plasmanylcholine ≈ phosphatidylcholine (19). Similarly, the rate constant of gramicidin-mediated K^+ ion flux across membranes composed of plasmenylcholine was substantially greater than that across bilayers composed of phosphatidylcholine (20). Collectively these studies demonstrate that ion transport, through both channel-mediated and carrier-mediated processes, occurs at substantially greater rates in biologic membranes composed of plasmalogen molecular species in comparison to diacyl phospholipid molecular species. These results could underlie the marked enrichment of plasmalogen molecular species in electrically active membranes.

Myocardial Phospholipase A₂ Is Calcium-Independent, Plasmalogen-Selective, ATP-Activated, and Physically Associated With Phosphofructokinase

Intracellular phospholipases A_2 comprise two functionally distinct types of enzymes, namely calcium-dependent phospholipase A_2 and calcium-independent phospholipase A_2. In the case of calcium-dependent phospholipases A_2, calcium facilitates hydrolysis of the *sn*-2 acyl linkage. Two major mechanisms account for the calcium dependence of these phospholipases. First, calcium can play a role in the polarization of the *sn*-2 carbonyl bond during catalysis, facilitating flux through the transition state during enzyme-catalyzed hydrolysis. Alternatively, calcium can facilitate the association of enzyme with the membrane interface to promote the formation of a productive complex. In sharp contrast to the phospholipases that possess an obligatory dependence on calcium ion for activity, calcium-independent phospholipases A_2 hydrolyze phospholipids at maximal rates in the absence of calcium ion and neither require calcium as an obligatory component in the catalytic process nor utilize calcium to facilitate binding of enzyme to the phospholipid surface.

In myocardium, the overwhelming majority of intracellular phospholipase A_2 activity is due to a calcium-independent phospholipase A_2, which was first described in 1985 (21). Based on the demonstrated predominance of plasmalogen molecular species in critical subcellular loci in myocardium (i.e., sarcolemma), synthetic radiolabeled plasmenylcholine substrate was prepared (22) and utilized to identify an enzyme that could selectively cleave arachidonic acid from the *sn*-2 acyl position of plasmalogen substrate. Moreover, this enzyme also selectively hydrolyzed phospholipid substrates containing arachidonic acid at the *sn*-2 position in both plasmenylcholine and phosphatidylcholine substrates (23, 24). Although the enzyme was selective for the hydrolysis of plasmalogen substrate, it should be stressed that the enzyme can actively hydrolyze diacyl phospholipid substrates (i.e., phosphatidylcholine and phosphatidylethanolamine molecular species) containing arachidonic acid at the *sn*-2 position.

To gain insight into the molecular mechanisms responsible for this enzyme's plasmalogen and arachidonic acid selectivity, we purified it by sequential column chromatographies (25). During the course of this purification we unexpectively observed a high affinity of the enzyme (or the enzyme complex and its regulatory proteins) to ATP. Detailed kinetic analysis demonstrated that the interaction between the phospholipase A_2 catalytic complex and ATP resulted in both the activation of the initial rate of fatty acid release from the *sn*-2 position of plasmenylcholine substrate as well as the dramatic attenuation of thermal denaturation of this enzyme (26). We exploited the interaction of myocardial phospholipase A_2 with ATP by using an ATP affinity column as the critical step in the purification strategy. We purified myocardial phospholipase A_2 157,000-fold to apparent homogeneity, identifying a 40-kDa polypeptide that cochromatographed with enzymic activity.

During the course of the purification we demonstrated (again unexpectedly) that a portion ($\approx 0.01\%$) of myocardial phosphofructokinase cochromatographed with phospholipase A_2 activity (27). Furthermore, antibodies to phosphofructokinase could immunoprecipitate phospholipase A_2 catalytic activity (27). Moreover, affinity columns composed of phosphofructokinase selectively bound myocardial phospholipase A_2 catalytic activity. Collectively, these results demonstrated that a high-affinity interaction between myocardial phospholipase A_2 and an isoform of phosphofructokinase was present. The combined demonstration of the activation of this enzyme by ATP, the cochromatography of phospholipase A_2 activity with phosphofructokinase, and identification of the native molecular weight of the enzyme complex of 400 kDa by gel filtration chromatography collectively identified myocardial phospholipase A_2 as a catalytic complex that was responsive to intracellular alterations in ATP concentration. Through these results, a potential mechanism for the regulation of this enzyme—namely activation through increases in intracellular ATP concentration by accelerated glycolytic flux—was postulated and explored, as will be seen below.

The Coupling of Glycolysis and Phospholipolysis Mediated by Calcium-Independent Phospholipase A_2

Although the concomitant activations of glycolysis and phospholipolysis during ischemia were previously thought to represent independent phenomena, the demonstration that calcium-independent phospholipase A_2 exists as an ATP-activatable catalytic complex, composed of a regulatory tetrameric phosphofructokinase subunit and a catalytic subunit, provided the key to identify the biochemical mechanisms underlying electrophysiologic dysfunction and myocytic cellular necrosis during the ischemic process.

First, it is important to recognize that acute myocardial ischemia is accompanied by dramatic increases in the rate of glycolytic flux, due in large part to the glucose derived from the breakdown of glycogen storage depots. Previous studies have demonstrated the ischemia-induced translocation of glycolytic complexes to membrane loci in muscle cells. Indeed, we have demonstrated that phosphofructokinase translocates from the cytosolic compartment to a membrane-associated compartment during myocardial ischemia (28). Accordingly, it is intriguing to hypothesize that membranes destined for hydrolysis are targeted by the delivery of the phospholipase A_2 catalytic complex to the specific subcellular membrane loci where it can be activated by compartmentalized increases in glycolytically derived ATP. During physiologic conditions this system can function to coordinate high-energy phosphate metabolism with electromechanical coupling and glycolytic flux, thereby facilitating appropriate cellular adaptation. The benefits of anaerobic production of ATP in ischemic myocardium from substrate-level phosphorylation during glycolysis are evident from both theoretic and chemical perspectives. However, it is clear that this system was never designed to provide the sole source of high-energy phosphate metabolites during prolonged (i.e., >20 min) intervals. Thus, during the prolonged and unremitting activation of glycolysis during severe ischemic events, accelerated phospholipid hydrolysis can occur, leading to deleterious amounts of phospholipid hydrolysis, thereby precipitating sarcolemmal dysfunction with resultant electrophysiologic alterations and myocytic cellular necrosis.

The coupling of glycolysis and phospholipolysis has many implications in other aspects of cardiac function as well. For example, alterations in cardiac contractility during hemodynamic stress are accompanied by altered glycolytic flux, subsequent increases in glycolytically derived ATP in critical subcellular loci, and thus the likely activation of calcium-independent phospholipase A_2. The resultant release of arachidonic acid could modulate ion channel function, thereby facilitating appropriate cardiovascular adaptation to a changing hemodynamic milieu. We stress the fact that both ischemia and increased hemodynamic demand are accompanied by increases in glycolytic flux and substrate-level ATP production. Thus, while it initially appears paradoxic that calcium-independent phospholipase A_2 is activated during ischemia *in vivo* and by ATP *in vitro*, in reality, activation by ATP likely reflects the compartmentalized changes in the local concentrations of ATP derived from accelerated glycolytic flux during ischemia. Alternatively, rapid alterations in creatine phosphate concentration concomitant with ischemia are well known, and the possibility that such alterations can couple with phospholipase A_2 catalytic activity through local changes in ATP concentrations represents an attractive hypothesis.

The Regulation of Myocardial Phospholipase A_2 by Calmodulin

Since myocardial phospholipase A_2 neither requires calcium as an obligatory cofactor in catalysis nor employs calcium for membrane association, it has traditionally been assumed that calcium ion does not directly regulate the activity of this enzyme. These conclusions had implicitly assumed that no associated calcium-responsive regulatory proteins were complexed with myocardial phospholipase A_2. In previous studies, we demonstrated that myocardial phospholipase A_2 did not have an obligatory dependence on calcium ion for catalytic activity; indeed, calcium ion actually markedly inhibited myocardial phospholipase A_2 activity. Purification of myocardial phospholipase A_2 demonstrated that although crude cytosolic myocardial phospholipase A_2 was inhibited by calcium ion, the purified enzyme was not inhibited by calcium.

These results led to reconstitution experiments in which crude myocardial cytosol and the purified phospholipase A_2 were mixed to reconstitute calcium-dependent inhibition, demonstrating that cytosol contained a protein factor that, in the presence of calcium ion, could inhibit myocardial phospholipase A_2 activity. Purification of this calcium-dependent phospholipase A_2 inhibitory factor demonstrated its identity with calmodulin by multiple independent criteria, including Western blotting and precipitation of the regulatory factor with W-7 agarose beads, and by reconstitution of calcium-mediated phospholipase A_2 inhibition with authentic homogeneous calmodulin (29). Moreover, calcium-induced calmodulin-mediated inhibition of myocardial phospholipase A_2 was titrated by physiologic increments of calcium ion (29). The mechanism through which calmodulin regulated myocardial phospholipase A_2 activity was demonstrated by ternary complex affinity chromatography, which revealed that calmodulin-sepharose avidly bound myocardial phospholipase A_2 activity (29). Thus, direct calcium-regulated protein-protein interactions between myocardial phospholipase A_2 and calmodulin occur. Importantly, treatment of cultured A-10 muscle cells with three structurally disparate calmodulin antagonists (i.e., W-7, trifluoperazine, and calmidazolium) resulted in the rapid release of [^{3}H] arachidonic acid from prelabeled A-10 muscle cells that was entirely ablated by pretreatment of cultured cells with the mechanism-based inhibitor (*E*)-6-(bromomethylene)-3-(1-naphthalenyl)-2*H*-tetrahydropyran-2-one (29).

These results identify a novel regulatory mechanism in muscle cells, whereby phospholipase A_2 activity is rendered latent by complexation with calcium and calmodulin and can be released from this tonic inhibition by physiologic alterations in calcium concentration, which modulate the interaction between the phospholipase A_2 catalytic complex and calmodulin. These results provide the first fundamental link between calmodulin, calcium ion, and the major phospholipase A_2 activity in myocardium. The significance of this observation is that a phospholipase A_2 that is nominally "calcium-independent" can be modulated by calcium ion through the calcium regulatory protein calmodulin.

The demonstration of the physical association of calmodulin with myocardial phospholipase A_2 and its functional coupling to myocardial phospholipase A_2 activity has important implications in cardiac physiology. During the cardiac cycle, concentrations of calcium vary from 150 nM during diastole to 600 nM during systole. The electrophysiologically active membrane of myocytes is highly enriched in plasmalogen molecular species containing arachidonic acid. Nonesterified arachidonic acid, released by calcium-independent phospholipase A_2, is a potent modulator of ion channel function (7). Accordingly, cardiac cycle–dependent alterations in electrophysiologic properties can, in principle, be mediated by cycle-dependent alterations in phospholipase A_2-catalyzed liberation of arachidonic acid. Thus, the functional coupling of myocardial phospholipase A_2 activity to calcium ion can potentially modulate cardiac cycle–dependent alterations in cellular electrophysiologic properties.

Summary

During this brief discussion we emphasized the specialized role of plasmalogens in myocardial membrane structure and function, both as critical determinants of the physical properties of the sarcolemmal membrane and as a reservoir for arachidonic acid released by myocardial calcium-independent phospholipase A_2. The activation of calcium-independent phospholipase A_2 during ischemia, with its translocation to critical membrane loci, provides a mechanistic rationale potentially underlying electrophysiologic dysfunction in ischemic zones. During physiologic conditions, the coupling of phospholipolysis with glycolysis likely facilitates physiologic adaptation during altered hemodynamic demands, whereas during the unremitting increase in glycolytic flux present during ischemia, local increases in ATP can result in potentially lethal sarcolemmal phospholipid hydrolysis and membrane dysfunction. Finally, the importance of the physical association and functional coupling of calmodulin with phospholipase A_2 is stressed, both from the physiologic perspective of cardiac cycle–dependent alterations in phospholipase A_2 activity as well as from a pathophysiologic perspective whereby ischemia may result in the release of the tonic inhibition of the phospholipase A_2, leading to sarcolemmal phospholipid hydrolysis and membrane dysfunction.

References

1. Katz, A.M., and Messineo, F.C. (1981) Lipid-Membrane Interactions and the Pathogenesis of Ischemic Damage in the Myocardium, *Circ. Res. 48,* 1–16.

2. Brenner, R.R. (1984) Effect of Unsaturated Acids on Membrane Structure and Enzyme Kinetics, *Prog. Lipid Res. 23,* 69–96.

3. Gross, R.W. (1992) Myocardial Phospholipases A_2 and Their Membrane Substrates, *Trends Cardiovasc. Med. 2,* 115–121.

4. Chien, K.R., Sen, A., Reynolds, R., Chang, A., Kim, Y., Gunn, M.D., Buja, L.M., and Willerson, J.T. (1985) Release of Arachidonate from Membrane Phospholipids in Cultured Neonatal Rat Myocardial Cells During Adenosine Triphosphate Depletion, *J. Clin. Invest. 75,* 1770–1780.

5. Gross, R.W. (1995) Myocardial Phospholipase A_2, *J. Lipid Mediat. 12,* 131–137.

6. Weltzien, H.U. (1979) Cytolytic and Membrane-Perturbing Properties of Lysophosphatidylcholine, *Biochim. Biophys. Acta 559,* 259–287.

7. Gubitosi-Klug, R., Yu, S.P., Choi, D.W., and Gross, R.W. (1995) Concomitant Acceleration of the Activation and Inactivation Kinetics of the Human Delayed Rectifier K^+ Channel (Kv1.1) by Ca^{2+}-Independent Phospholipase A_2, *J. Biol. Chem. 270,* 2885–2888.

8. Briggs, M.M., and Lefkowitz, R.J. (1980) Parallel Modulation of Catecholamine Activation of Adenylate Cyclase and Formation of the High-Affinity Agonist-Receptor Complex in Turkey Erythrocyte Membranes by Temperature and cis-Vaccenic Acid, *Biochemistry 19,* 4461–4466.

9. Honoré, E., Barhanin, J., Attali, B., Lesage, F., and Lazdunski, M. (1994) External Blockade of the Major Cardiac Delayed-Rectifier K^+ Channel (Kv1.5) by Polyunsaturated Fatty Acids, *Proc. Natl. Acad. Sci. USA 91,* 1937–1944.

10. Feulgen, R., and Voit, K. (1924) Über einen weitverbreiteten festen Aldehyd. Seine Entstehung aus einer Vorstufe, sein mikrochemischer und mikroskopisch-chemischer Nachweis und die Wege zu seiner präparativen Darstellung, *Pflugers Arch. Gesamte Physiol. Menschen Tiere 206,* 389–410.

11. Pak, J.H., Bork, V.P., Norberg, R.E., Creer, M.H., Wolf, R.A., and Gross, R.W. (1987) Disparate Molecular Dynamics of Plasmenylcholine and Phosphatidylcholine Bilayers, *Biochemistry 26,* 4824–4830.

12. Han, X., and Gross, R.W. (1990) Plasmenylcholine and Phosphatidylcholine Membrane Bilayers Possess Distinct Conformational Motifs, *Biochem. 26,* 4992–4996.

13. Han, X., Chen, X., and Gross, R.W. (1991) Chemical and Magnetic Inequivalence of Glycerol Protons in Individual Subclasses of Choline Glycerophospholipids: Implications for Subclass-Specific Changes in Membrane Conformational States, *J. Am. Chem. Soc. 113,* 7104–7109.

14. Han, X., and Gross, R.W. (1991) Proton Nuclear Magnetic Resonance Studies on the Molecular Dynamics of Plasmenylcholine/Cholesterol and Phosphatidylcholine/Cholesterol Bilayers, *Biochem. Biophys. Acta 1063,* 129–136.

15. Han, X., and Gross, R.W. (1992) Nonmonotonic Alterations in the Fluorescence Anisotropy of Polar Head Group Labeled Fluorophores During the Lamellar to Hexagonal Phase Transition of Phospholipids, *Biophys. J. Biophys. Soc. 63,* 309–316.

16. Gross, R.W. (1984) High Plasmalogen and Arachidonic Acid Content of Canine Myocardial Sarcolemma: A Fast Atom Bombardment Mass Spectroscopic and Gas Chromatography-Mass Spectroscopic Characterization, *Biochemistry 23*, 158–165.

17. Gross, R.W. (1985) Identification of Plasmalogen as the Major Phospholipid Constituent of Cardiac Sarcoplasmic Reticulum, *Biochemistry 24*, 1662–1668.

18. Chen, X., Han, X., and Gross, R.W. (1993) Dynamics of Binary Mixtures of Plasmenylcholine/Arachidonic Acid and Phosphatidylcholine/Arachidonic Acid—A Study Using Fluorescence and NMR Spectroscopy, *Biochim. Biophys. Acta 1149*, 241–248.

19. Chen, X., and Gross, R.W. (1994) Phospholipid Subclass-Specific Alterations in the Kinetics of Ion Transport across Biologic Membranes, *Biochemistry 33*, 13769–13774.

20. Chen, X., and Gross, R.W. (1995) Potassium Flux through Gramicidin Ion Channels Is Augmented in Vesicles Comprising Plasmenylcholine: Correlations Between Gramicidin Conformation and Function in Chemically Distinct Host Bilayer Matrices. *Biochemistry 22*, 1756–1764.

21. Wolf, R.A., and Gross, R.W. (1985) Identification of Neutral Active Phospholipase C Which Hydrolyzes Choline Glycerophospholipids and Plasmalogen Selective Phospholipase A_2 in Canine Myocardium, *J. Biol. Chem. 260*, 7295–7303.

22. Wolf, R.A., and Gross, R.W. (1985) Semi-Synthetic Approach for the Preparation of Homogeneous Plasmenylethanolamine Utilizing Phospholipase D from *Streptomyces chromofuscus*, *J. Lipid Res. 26*, 629–633.

23. Hazen, S.L., and Gross, R.W. (1991) Human Myocardial Cytosolic Calcium-Independent Phospholipase A_2 Is Modulated by ATP: Concordant ATP-Induced Alterations in Enzyme Kinetics and Mechanism-Based Inhibition, *Biochem. J. 280*, 581–587.

24. Hazen, S.L., and Gross, R.W. (1992) Identification and Characterization of Human Myocardial Phospholipase A_2 from Transplant Recipients Suffering from End Stage Ischemic Heart Disease, *Circ. Res. 70*, 487–495.

25. Hazen, S.L., Stuppy, R.J., and Gross, R.W. (1990) Purification and Characterization of Canine Myocardial Cytosolic Phospholipase A_2: A Calcium-Independent Phospholipase with Absolute *sn*-2 Regiospecificity for Diradyl Glycerophospholipids, *J. Biol. Chem. 265*, 10622–10630.

26. Hazen, S.L., and Gross, R.W. (1991) ATP-Dependent Regulation of Rabbit Myocardial Cytosolic Calcium-Independent Phospholipase A_2, *J. Biol. Chem. 266*, 14526–14534.

27. Hazen, S.L., and Gross, R.W. (1993) The Specific Association of a Phosphofructokinase Isoform with Myocardial Calcium-Independent Phospholipase A_2: Implications for the Coordinated Regulation of Phospholipolysis and Glycolysis, *J. Biol. Chem. 268*, 9892–9900.

28. Hazen, S.L., Wolf, M.J., Ford, D.A., and Gross, R.W. (1994) The Rapid and Reversible Association of Phosphofructokinase with Myocardial Membranes, *FEBS Lett. 339*, 213–216.

29. Wolf, M.J., and Gross, R.W. (1994) The Calcium-Dependent Association and Functional Coupling of Calmodulin with Myocardial Phospholipase A_2, *J. Biol. Chem. 271*, 20989–20994.

Chapter 11

An Isoform of Intracellular Platelet-Activating Factor (PAF) Acetylhydrolase and Its Relationship to Miller-Dieker Syndrome

Hiroyuki Arai, Mitsuharu Hattori, Junken Aoki, and Keizo Inoue

Department of Health Chemistry, Faculty of Pharmaceutical Sciences,
The University of Tokyo, Hongo 7-3-1, Bunkyo-ku, Tokyo 113, Japan

Platelet-Activating Factor Acetylhydrolase—Its Discovery and Classification

Platelet-activating factor (PAF) is one of the most potent lipid messenger molecules implicated in a variety of physiological events. The acetyl moiety at the *sn*-2 position of its glycerol backbone is indispensable for its biological activity, and its deacetylation induces loss of activity. Deacetylation reaction is catalyzed by PAF acetylhydrolase (PAH-AH), a member of the phospholipase A_2 family (1). The PAF-AH activity was first described in 1980 by Farr et al. (2). Subsequently, Blank et al. reported that this enzyme was distributed ubiquitously in mammalian tissues and blood and that it was specific for deacetylation of phospholipids (3). They also suggested that the PAF-AH activities of plasma and of kidney soluble fraction would be due to different proteins, because only the latter was affected by treatment with proteases (4). From then on, a series of biochemical and enzymological characterization revealed that there were two types in PAF-AH—intracellular (tissue) and extracellular (plasma)—based on their sensitivities to some inhibitors, their molecular weights, and their hydrolytic activities against methylated analogs of PAF (5–7). The extracellular type of PAF-AH was purified from human plasma in 1987 by Stafforini et al. (8, 9), who extensively characterized the protein (10–14) and cloned its cDNA in 1995 (15). Recently it has become clear that there is no other protein in human plasma that catalyzes deacetylation of PAF, since a genetic deficit of this protein leads to lack of PAF-AH activity in plasma (16,17). Stafforini et al. also reported occurrences of PAF-AH activity in human erythrocytes (18) and partial purification of the enzyme (19).

We found that PAF-AH activity in bovine brain soluble fraction was chromatographically separated into three distinct fractions, designated Ia, Ib, and II (20). Similar results were obtained when bovine kidney, bovine liver, and rat brain were used as starting materials (20, 21, and our unpublished observations), suggesting that there were at least three isoforms of PAF-AH within mammalian tissues. None of them were thought to be of lysosomal origin, as they exhibited pH optima in the neutral to mild alkaline region (20). We purified the isoform Ib from bovine brain soluble fraction (20) and isoform II from bovine liver (21). Also, we cloned their cDNAs (22–25) and revealed that isoforms Ib and II had totally different structures. In this chapter, we focus on the structure of mammalian intracellular PAF-AH isoform Ib and its implication in neuronal development.

Structure of Intracellular PAF Acetylhydrolase Isoform Ib

Intracellular PAF-AH isoform Ib consists of three heterologous subunits originally designated α, β, and γ. We now call these β, α_2, and α_1, respectively, since the overall structure of the enzyme is similar to that of trimeric G-protein (Fig. 11.1 and Table 11.1) (26). Their molecular weights, as estimated by sodium dodecylsulfate gel electrophoresis (SDS-PAGE), are 45, 30, and 29 kDa, respectively. Since the apparent molecular mass of the native form calculated from a gel filtration column chromatography was about 100 kDa, these subunits are likely to be present in a relative stoichiometry of one copy each (20), which has also been confirmed by cross-linking experiments (24).

The enzyme is strongly inhibited by diisopropyl fluorophosphate (DFP) (20), an active serine modifier, and a labeling experiment using ^{3}H-DFP showed that both the α_1 (formerly γ) and α_2 (formerly β) subunits have an active serine residue (24). When purified isoform Ib was applied to Heparin-Sepharose or a sulfated cellulose column chromatography under mild acidic conditions, most of its activity passed through the column. Both the α_1 and α_2 subunits comigrated precisely with the enzyme activity (i.e., passed through the column), whereas the β (formerly α) subunit was adsorbed to the column and recovered by NaCl elution. The α_1/α_2 heterodimer still exhibited full enzymatic activity, and neither its K_m nor its V_{max} was changed when assayed *in vitro* with PAF as a substrate (23). These observations indicated that the β subunit may function as a "regulatory unit."

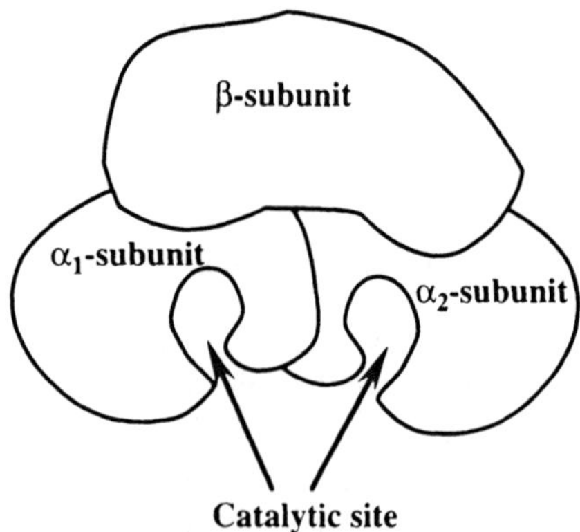

Fig. 11.1. Structure of PAF-AH Ib.

TABLE 11.1
Nomenclature and Molecular Weights of PAF-AH Ib Subunits

New name	Former name	Molecular weight (kDa on SDS-PAGE)
β subunit	α subunit	45
α_2 subunit	β subunit	30
α_1 subunit	γ subunit	29

cDNA cloning of the α_1 and α_2 subunits revealed that their amino acid sequences are homologous (63.2%) with each other (22,24), but that they are homologous to no other proteins reported so far. Conserved residues were distributed almost all over the sequence. Expression experiments in *E. coli* showed that each of them forms homodimers when overexpressed and that both of them have PAF-AH activity that is comparable to that of the native enzyme (24).

As previously mentioned, this enzyme is strongly inhibited by DFP, suggesting that it is a member of the serine esterase family (27). However, the α_1 and α_2 subunits do not have a consensus sequence of serine esterase surrounding the active serine residue: Gly–Xaa–Active Ser–Xaa–Gly. Therefore, we determined the active serine residue of these subunits (Ser47 and Ser48, respectively, of the α_1 and α_2 subunits) (22, 24). The second residue from the active serine residue is Val, where Gly is conserved in almost all serine esterases. The present enzyme has another unique characteristic: In the catalytic subunits of PAF-AH Ib the active serine residues occur very early (i.e., close to the N-terminal end), whereas in most other serine esterases the active serine residue is 100 to 250 residues away from the N-terminal end. These facts suggest that the catalytic subunits of intracellular PAF-AH isoform Ib have a novel fold as a serine esterase. Indeed, we recently succeeded in revealing the 3D structure of the homodimer of the α_1 subunit by X-ray crystallography (26) and found that its structure is not similar to that of any known serine esterase. Instead, its 3D structure is strikingly similar to that of p21[Ras] and also to that of the GTP-binding domain of the α subunit of trimeric G protein.

In addition, the β subunit is homologous to the β subunit of G protein in that it has seven WD repeats (Fig. 11.2), which are often found in proteins that function through interaction with other protein components (28,29). Thus, we may say that PAF-AH Ib is essentially a G protein-like trimer. It is probable that binding of PAF to this trimer triggers conformational changes in the catalytic dimer that result in the release of the β subunit. For this reason we changed the names of the subunits to correspond to the nomenclature of a trimeric G protein.

The amino acid sequence of the β subunit was also found to match that of the product of the causative gene (*LIS-1*) for human Miller-Dieker syndrome (MDS) (23). Of the 410 amino acid residues in bovine β subunit, 409 are identical to those in the human *LIS-1* protein, indicating that the *LIS-1* product could be a human homolog of the β subunit of bovine brain PAF-AH isoform Ib.

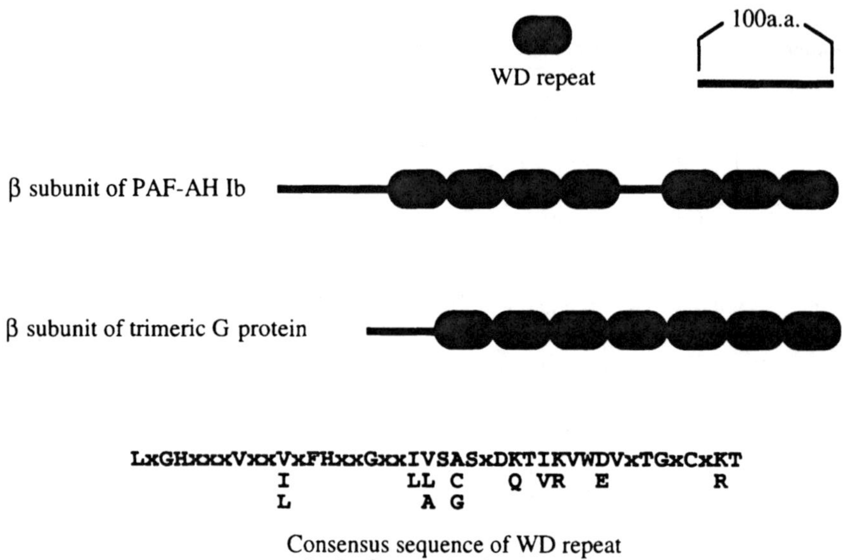

Fig. 11.2. WD repeat in the β subunit of PAF-AH Ib and its comparison with that of the β subunit of trimeric G protein.

Miller-Dieker Syndrome and PAF Metabolism

MDS is a rare disorder (about one or two per million live births) that consists of brain malformation, manifested by a smooth cerebral surface (lissencephaly); a characteristic facial appearance; and often other abnormalities (30–32). The brain malformation results from arrest of neuronal migration in the cerebral cortex and elsewhere at about 10–14 weeks of fetal development. Although this disorder had been thought to be an autosomal recessive one, cytogenetic studies by Ledbetter et al. demonstrated that microdeletion of chromosome 17p13.3 is the cause of MDS and that this can result even from *de novo* events (33,34). The causative gene in 17p13.3 (*LIS-1*) was then identified through genetic techniques by Reiner et al., who assumed that the *LIS-1* protein could be involved in signal transduction, because it had the WD repeat (35).

We found that the *LIS-1* protein is a human homolog of the β subunit of bovine intracellular PAF-AH Ib, raising the possibility that this heterotrimeric enzyme plays an essential role during brain development. As summarized in Table 11.2, several reports suggest that PAF can serve as a transmitter in the nervous system. Although the β subunit has no appreciable effect on the enzymatic activity of the α_1/α_2 subunits *in vitro*, we suppose that localization and/or activity *in vivo* of PAF-AH Ib would be regulated through the β subunit. Then the concentration of PAF would be maintained within a certain range, which would be important for normal development.

TABLE 11.2
Observations That Suggest Roles of PAF in the Nervous System

Observation	Reference
PAF induces differentiation of cultured neuronal cells.	37
PAF is produced in nervous tissues in response to stimuli.	38–41
Neurite outgrowth is modulated by PAF.	42
The PAF receptor is present in the central nervous system.	43
Neuronal cells increase PAF production when they begin to mature and form synaptic-like junctions.	44
PAF can serve as a retrograde messenger in long-term potentiation.	45
PAF produces neuronal growth cone collapse.	46

In order to obtain a clue to understand the precise function of this enzyme during brain development, we investigated whether the subunits are coexpressed in the murine developing and adult brain (36). It is shown by *in situ* hybridization that all the subunits' genes are coexpressed in developing neuronal tissues. Furthermore, the expression pattern is consistent with the neuronal migration defects seen in MDS: Regions containing migrating neurons, such as the developing cerebral and cerebellar cortices, express these genes at a particularly high level. On the other hand, in the adult brain, mRNA of the β (α) and α_2 (β) subunits continue to be coexpressed at high levels whereas that of the α_1 (γ) subunit is greatly decreased, suggesting that the heterotrimer disappears in adult brains. Further studies, using antibodies against each subunit, would be needed to determine the precise expression pattern.

Summary

We have studied the structure and function of intracellular PAF-AHs. PAF-AH Ib, a heterotrimeric enzyme, has a unique structure with two catalytic units (the α_1 and α_2 subunits) and one noncatalytic unit (the β subunit). The role of the β subunit is presently unknown, but a hemizygous deletion of the gene for the β subunit results in MDS, a brain malformation resulting from abnormal neuronal migration. Although the molecular mechanism of neuronal migration is not well understood, PAF-AH, and possibly PAF, may play a crucial role in the process.

References

1. Dennis, E.A. (1994) Diversity of Group Types, Regulation, and Function of Phospholipase A2, *J. Biol. Chem. 269*, 175–178.
2. Farr, R.S., Cox, C.P., Wardlow, M.L., and Jorgensen, R. (1980) Preliminary Studies of an Acid-Labile Factor (ALF) in Human Sera That Inactivates Platelet-Activating Factor (PAF), *Clin. Immunol. Immunopathol. 15*, 318–330.

3. Blank, M.L., Lee, T-C., Fitzgerald, V., and Snyder, F. (1981)A Specific Acetylhydrolase for 1-Alkyl-2-acetyl-*sn*-glycero-3-phosphocholine (A Hypotensive and Platelet-Activating Lipid), *J. Biol. Chem. 256*, 175–178.

4. Blank, M.L., Hall, M.N., Cress, A.E., and Snyder, F. (1983) Inactivation of 1-Alkyl-2-acetyl-*sn*-glycero-3-phosphocholine by a Plasma Acetylhydrolase: Higher Activities in Hypertensive Rats, *Biochem. Biophys. Res. Commun. 113*, 666–671.

5. Wardlow, M.L., Cox, C.P., Meng, K.E., Greene, D.E., and Farr, R.S. (1986) Substrate Specificity and Partial Characterization of the PAF-acylhydrolase in Human Serum that Rapidly Inactivates Platelet-Activating Factor, *J. Immunol. 136*, 3441–3446.

6. Yanoshita, R., Kudo, I., Ikizawa, K., Chang, H.W., Kobayashi, S., Ohno, M., Nojima, S., and Inoue, K. (1988) Hydrolysis of Platelet Activating Factor and Its Methylated Analogs by Acetylhydrolases, *J. Biochem. (Tokyo) 103*, 815–819.

7. Stafforini, D.M., Prescott, S.M., Zimmerman, G.A. and McIntyre, T.M. (1991) Platelet-Activating Factor Acetylhydrolase Activity in Human Tissues and Blood Cells, *Lipids 26*, 979–985.

8. Stafforini, D.M., McIntyre, T.M., Carter, M.E., and Prescott, S.M. (1987) Human Plasma Platelet-Activating Factor Acetylhydrolase. Association with Lipoprotein Particles and Role in the Degradation of Platelet-Activating Factor, *J. Biol. Chem. 262*, 4215–4222.

9. Stafforini, D.M., Prescott, S.M., and McIntyre, T.M. (1987) Human Plasma Platelet-Activating Factor Acetylhydrolase. Purification and Properties, *J. Biol. Chem. 262*, 4223–4230.

10. Stremler, K.E., Stafforini, D.M., Prescott, S.M., Zimmerman, G.A., and McIntyre, T.M. (1989) An Oxidized Derivative of Phosphatidylcholine Is a Substrate for the Platelet-Activating Factor Acetylhydrolase from Human Plasma, *J. Biol. Chem. 264*, 5331–5334.

11. Stafforini, D.M., Carter, M.E., Zimmerman, G.A., McIntyre, T.M., and Prescott, S.M. (1989) Lipoproteins Alter the Catalytic Behavior of the Platelet-Activating Factor Acetylhydrolase in Human Plasma, *Proc. Natl. Acad. Sci. USA 86*, 2393–2397.

12. Stremler, K.E., Stafforini, D.M., Prescott, S.M., and McIntyre, T.M. (1991) Human Plasma Platelet-Activating Factor Acetylhydrolase. Oxidatively Fragmented Phospholipids as Substrates, *J. Biol. Chem. 266*, 11095–11103.

13. Smiley, P.L., Stremler, K.E., Prescott, S.M., Zimmerman, G.A., and McIntyre, T.M. (1991) Oxidatively Fragmented Phosphatidylcholines Activate Human Neutrophils Through the Receptor for Platelet-Activating Factor, *J. Biol. Chem. 266*, 11104–11110.

14. Tarbet, E.B., Stafforini, D.M., Elstad, M.R., Zimmerman, G.A., McIntyre, T.M., and Prescott, S.M. (1991) Liver Cells Secrete the Plasma Form of Platelet-Activating Factor Acetylhydrolase, *J. Biol. Chem. 266*, 16667–16673.

15. Tjoelker, L.W., Wilder, C., Eberhardt, C., Stafforini, D.M., Dietsch, G., Schimpf, B., Hooper, S., Trong, H.L., Cousens, L.S., Zimmerman, G.A., Yamada, Y., McIntyre, T.M., Prescott, S.M., and Gray, P.W. (1995) Anti-inflammatory Properties of a Platelet-Activating Factor Acetylhydrolase, *Nature 374*, 549–553.

16. Miwa, M., Miyake, T., Yamanaka, T., Sugatani, J., Suzuki, Y., Sakata, S., Araki, Y., and Matsumoto, M. (1988) Characterization of Serum Platelet-Activating Factor (PAF) Acetylhydrolase. Correlation Between Deficiency of Serum PAF Acetylhydrolase and Respiratory Symptoms in Asthmatic Children, *J. Clin. Invest. 82*, 1983–1991.

17. Stafforini, D.M., Prescott, S.M., Zimmerman, G.A., and McIntyre, T.M. (1996) Mammalian Platelet-Activating Factor Acetylhydrolases, *Biochim. Biophys. Acta 1301*, 161–173.

18. Stafforini, D.M., Prescott, S.M., and McIntyre, T.M. (1991) Platelet-Activating Factor Acetylhydrolase in Human Erythrocytes, *Meths. Enzymol. 197*, 411–425.

19. Stafforini, D.M., Rollins, E.N., Prescott, S.M., and McIntyre, T.M. (1993) The Platelet-Activating Factor Acetylhydrolase from Human Erythrocytes. Purification and Properties, *J. Biol. Chem. 268*, 3857–3865.

20. Hattori, M., Arai, H., and Inoue, K. (1993) Purification and Characterization of Bovine Brain Platelet-Activating Factor Acetylhydrolase, *J. Biol. Chem. 268*, 18748–18753.

21. Hattori, K., Hattori, M., Adachi, H., Tsujimoto, M., Arai, H., and Inoue, K. (1995) Purification and Characterization of Platelet-Activating Factor Acetylhydrolase II from Bovine Liver Cytosol, *J. Biol. Chem. 270*, 22308–22313.

22. Hattori, M., Adachi, H., Tsujimoto, M., Arai, H., and Inoue, K. (1994) The Catalytic Subunit of Bovine Brain Platelet-Activating Factor Acetylhydrolase Is a Novel Type of Serine Esterase, *J. Biol Chem. 269*, 23150–23155.

23. Hattori, M., Adachi, H., Tsujimoto, M., Arai, H., and Inoue, K. (1994) Miller-Dieker Lissencephaly Gene Encodes a Subunit of Brain Platelet-Activating Factor Acetylhydrolase, *Nature 370*, 216–218.

24. Hattori, M., Adachi, H., Aoki, J., Tsujimoto, M., Arai, H., and Inoue, K. (1995) Cloning and Expression of a cDNA Encoding the Beta-Subunit (30-kDa Subunit) of Bovine Brain Platelet-Activating Factor Acetylhydrolase, *J. Biol Chem. 270*, 31345–31352.

25. Hattori, K., Adachi, H., Matsuzawa, A., Yamamoto, K., Tsujimoto, M., Aoki, J., Hattori, M., Arai, H., and Inoue, K. (1996) cDNA Cloning and Expression of Intracellular Platelet-Activating Factor (PAF) Acetylhydrolase II. Its Homology with Plasma PAF Acetylhydrolase, *J. Biol. Chem. 271*, 33032–33038.

26. Ho, Y.S., Swenson, L., Derewenda, U., Dauter, Z., Hattori, M., Aoki, J., Arai, H., Inoue, K., and Derewenda, Z.S. (1997) Brain Acetylhydrolase That Inactivates Platelet-Activating Factor is a G-Protein-Like Trimer, *Nature 385*, 89–93.

27. Brenner, S. (1988) The Molecular Evolution of Genes and Proteins: A Tale of Two Serines, *Nature 334*, 5463–5467.

28. Van der Voorn, L., and Ploegh, H.L. (1992) The WD-40 Repeat, *FEBS Lett. 307*, 131–134.

29. Neer, E.J., Scmidt, C.J., Nambudripad, R., Smith, T.F. (1994) The Ancient Regulatory-Protein Family of WD-Repeat Proteins, *Nature 371*, 297–300.

30. de Rijk-van Andel, J.F., Arts, W.F.M., Hofman, A., Ataal, A., and Niermeijar, M.F. (1991) *Neuroepidermiol. 10*, 200–204.

31. Dobyns, W.B., Curry, C.J.R., Hoyme, H.E., Turlington, L., and Ledbetter, D.H. (1991) *Am. J. Hum. Genet. 48*, 584–594.

32. Dobyns, W.B., Reiner, O., Carrozzo, R., and Ledbetter, D.H. (1993) *J. Am. Med. Assoc. 270*, 2838–2842.

33. Stratton, R.F., Dobyns, W.B., Airhart, S.D., and Ledbetter, D.H. (1984) *Hum. Genet. 67*, 193–200.

34. Greenberg, F., Stratton, R.F., Lockhart, L.H., Elder, F.F.B., Dobyns, W.B., Ledbetter, D.H. (1986) *Am. J. Med. Genet. 23*, 853–859.

35. Reiner, O., Carrozzo, R., Shen, Y., Wehnert, M., Faustinella, F., Dobyns, W.B., Caskey, C.T., and Ledbetter, D.H. (1993) *Nature 364*, 717–721.

36. Albrecht, U., Abu-Issa, R., Ratz, B., Hattori, M., Aoki, J., Arai, H., Inoue, K., and Eichele, G. (1996) *Dev. Biol.*, in press.

37. Kornecki, E., and Ehrlich, Y.H. (1988) *Science 240*, 1792–1794.

38. Kumar, R., Harvey, A.K., Kester, M., Hanahan, D.J., and Olson, M.S. (1988) *Biochim. Biophys. Acta 963*, 375–383.

39. Sogos, V., Bussolino, F., Pilia, E., Torelli, S., and Gremo, F. (1990) *J. Neurosci. Res. 27*, 706–711.

40. Yue, T-L., Lysko, P.G., and Feuerstein, G. (1990) *J. Neurochem. 54*, 1809–1811.

41. Marcheselli, V.L. and Bazan, N.G. (1994) *J. Neurosci. Res. 37*, 54–61.

42. Herrick-Davis, K., Camussi, G., Bussolino, F., and Baglioni, C. (1991) *J. Biol. Chem. 266*, 18620–18625.

43. Bito, H., Nakamura, M., Honda, Z., Izumi, T., Iwatsubo, T., Seyama, Y., Ogura, A., Kudo, Y., and Shimizu, T. (1992) *Neuron 9*, 285–294.

44. Francescangeli, E., Freysz, L., Dreyfus, H., Boila, A., and Goracci, G. (1993) in *Phospholipids and Signal Transmission*, Massarelli, R., Horrocks, L.A., Kanfer, J.N., and Loffelholz, K., eds., Springer-Verlag, Berlin, 373–385.

45. Kato, K., Clark, G.D., Bazen, N.G., and Zorumski, C.F. (1994) *Nature 367*, 175–179.

46. Clark, G.D., McNeil, R.S., Bix, G.J., and Swann, J.W. (1995) *NeuroReport 6*, 2569–2575.

Chapter 12

Homocysteine and Vascular Disease: The Role of Folate, Choline, and Lipoproteins in Homocysteine Metabolism

Kilmer S. McCully

Pathology and Laboratory Medicine Service, Veterans Affairs Medical Center, Providence, RI

Discovery of the Atherogenic Effect of Homocysteine

Homocystinuria is an inherited disease caused by homozygous deficiencies of one of three enzymes of homocysteine metabolism: cystathionine synthase, methyltetrahydrofolate homocysteine methyl transferase, or methylenetetrahydrofolate reductase. In the most common form of homocystinuria, deficiency of cystathionine synthase causes increased blood levels of homocystine, protein-bound homocysteine, and homocysteine cysteine disulfide because the transsulfuration pathway to cystathionine is inhibited. Failure of cystathionine synthesis from homocysteine leads to increased blood methionine levels and decreased formation of cysteine, cysteine sulfinic acid, and sulfate. Cases of cystathionine synthase deficiency have greatly increased risk of thrombosis and arterial vascular lesions (1–4).

The atherogenic effect of homocysteine was discovered by observation of arteriosclerotic lesions in a child with homocystinuria, cystathioninuria, and methylmalonic aciduria caused by deficiency of methyltetrahydrofolate homocysteine methyl transferase (5,6). In this disease, blood levels of homocystine, homocysteine cysteine disulfide, and cystathionine are elevated and blood levels of methionine are low. Arteriosclerotic lesions are attributed to a direct damaging effect of homocysteine on the cells and tissues of artery walls in methyl transferase deficiency and cystathionine synthase deficiency, because elevation of blood homocysteine is the only metabolic abnormality shared by these two diseases.

The conclusion that homocysteine is atherogenic is supported by the finding of arteriosclerotic lesions in a child with methylenetetrahydrofolate reductase deficiency (7). In this disease the blood homocysteine level is elevated because of decreased formation of methyltetrahydrofolate and decreased methylation of homocysteine to methionine by methylcobalamin. Thus arteriosclerotic lesions are attributable to hyperhomocysteinemia in the three principal forms of homocystinuria, each caused by inherited deficiency of a different enzyme of homocysteine metabolism, as illustrated in Fig. 12.1.

Parenteral administration of homocysteine in its reactive anhydride form (homocysteine thiolactone) in rabbits and baboons causes arteriosclerotic plaques that resemble the lesions found in human cases of homocystinuria (8,9). The plaques of

K.S. McCully

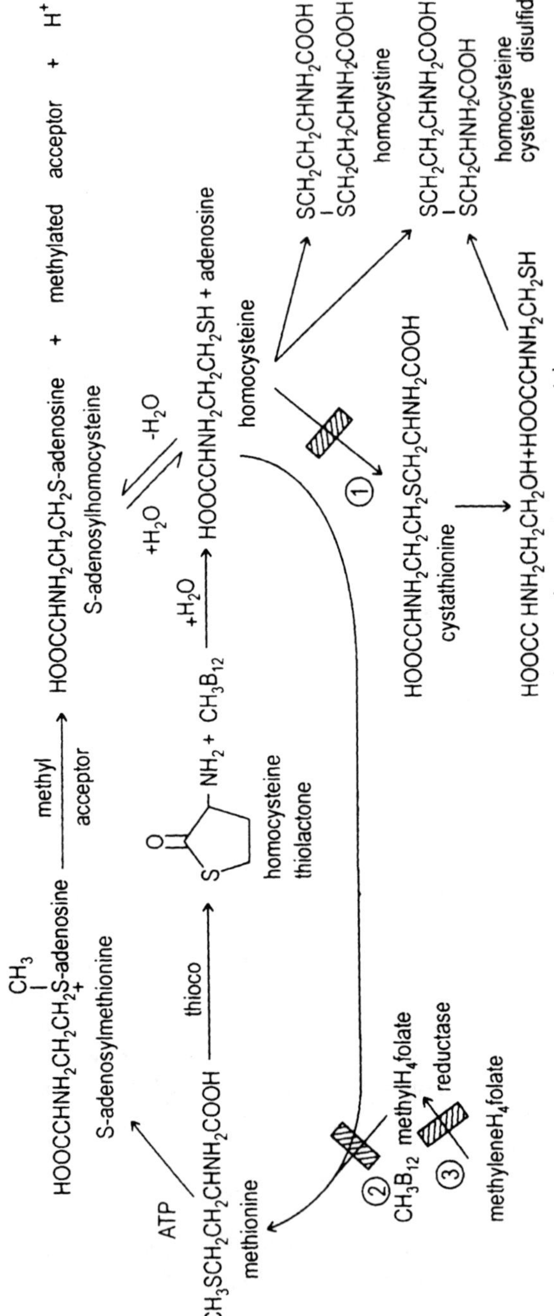

Fig. 12.1. Inherited disorders of homocysteine metabolism. Genetic deficiencies of cystathionine synthase (enzyme 1), methyltetrahydrofolate homocysteine methyl transferase (enzyme 2), or methylenetetrahydrofolate reductase (enzyme 3) produce homocystinuria and hyperhomocysteinemia.

the aorta and the coronary, renal, cerebral, and peripheral arteries consist of deposits of sulfated glycosaminoglycans, hyperplastic smooth-muscle cells, degenerative elastica interna, calcification, and fibrosis. If homocystine is oxidized with hydrogen peroxide and fed in a synthetic diet, or if methionine is converted to S-methylhomocysteine thiolactone and fed in a synthetic diet, prominent fibrous arteriosclerotic plaques are observed in rabbits (10). If the synthetic diet contains cholesterol (8) or butter, and the animals are given the homocysteine thiolactonyl derivatives thioretinamide or thioretinaco, fibrolipid plaques are observed (11). Corn oil in the synthetic diet in place of butter prevents hyperhomocysteinemia and fibrolipid plaques.

High doses of parenteral homocysteine thiolactone in rabbits cause venous thrombosis, pulmonary embolism, and pulmonary infarction that are prevented by parenteral pyridoxine (10,12). Chronic pyridoxine deficiency causes arteriosclerotic plaques in monkeys (13) and pigs (14). The preventive effect of pyridoxine against thrombosis and arteriosclerosis in these animal models is attributable to prevention of hyperhomocysteinemia because of increased conversion of homocysteine to cystathionine. Although a few studies have been inconclusive, most reports have concluded that homocysteine is atherogenic in experimental pyridoxine deficiency or in experimental hyperhomocysteinemia.

The first human study to demonstrate abnormal homocysteine metabolism in vascular-disease patients showed that the blood level of homocysteine cysteine disulfide becomes more highly elevated in these patients than in controls following an oral dose of methionine (15). More recently, blood homocysteine levels have been found in a number of studies to be elevated in patients with coronary, cerebral, or peripheral arteriosclerosis (16). Hyperhomocysteinemia is now generally accepted as a major independent risk factor for arteriosclerosis. A recent large-scale cross-sectional analysis of a population at risk showed that hyperhomocysteinemia is correlated with known risk factors for vascular disease, including male sex, postmenopausal status, smoking, lack of exercise, elevated blood cholesterol, and elevated blood pressure (17).

Genetic factors, especially heterozygous thermolabile methylenetetrahydrofolate reductase, have been shown to increase risk for hyperhomocysteinemia and for coronary heart disease in the general population. In a study of French Canadians the allele frequency of this abnormal enzyme was demonstrated in 38% of the population by techniques of molecular biology (18). Population studies of the frequency of cystathionine synthase deficiency by oral methionine tolerance testing and by enzymatic analysis of cultured fibroblasts have suggested that as many as 32% of early-onset arteriosclerotic disease cases may be heterozygous for this enzyme (19). However, more recent studies of heterozygosity for cystathionine synthase deficiency, using allele analysis by techniques of molecular genetics, have failed to associate heterozygosity for this abnormal enzyme with risk of coronary heart disease (20). The overall incidence of genetic factors predisposing to hyperhomocysteinemia has been estimated to be approximately one-third of cases of early-onset arteriosclerosis (21).

Dietary factors, including deficiencies of folate, pyridoxine, and cobalamin, were found to be associated with low blood levels of these micronutrients, hyperhomocysteinemia (22), and narrowing of carotid arteries (23) in a study of elderly participants in the Framingham Heart Study. In a prospective study of 14,000 US physicians, the risk of myocardial infarction was found to be increased threefold among participants with hyperhomocysteinemia (24). No prospective prevention trials have been completed to show whether increasing the intake of vitamin B_6, folic acid, or vitamin B_{12} from dietary or supplemental sources affects risk of arteriosclerosis. Recent studies have shown increased risk of hyperhomocysteinemia and coronary heart disease to be associated with deficiency of plasma pyridoxal phosphate (25) or plasma folate (26). A retrospective study showed that moderately high doses of vitamin B_6 given for carpal tunnel syndrome reduced the risk of angina pectoris and myocardial infarction by 73% and increased apparent longevity by 7–17 years (27). These various human studies have fulfilled the prediction that hyperhomocysteinemia would prove to be a major factor in the pathogenesis of arteriosclerosis in the general population (5,10,28). This discovery offers new strategies and opportunities for prevention and treatment of the disease (29).

Control of Homocysteine Metabolism

Methionine is converted in the liver to adenosyl methionine, a major methyl donor in transmethylation reactions. Following transfer of the methyl group to an acceptor molecule, the resulting adenosyl homocysteine is reversibly converted to adenosine and free homocysteine by adenosyl homocysteine hydrolase, an enzyme that thermodynamically favors synthesis of adenosyl homocysteine. Adenosyl methionine is an allosteric activator of cystathionine synthase and inhibitor of methylenetetrahydrofolate reductase, regulating the synthesis of homocysteine by activation of the transsulfuration pathway and by inhibition of the remethylation pathway (30). This regulatory control of homocysteine homeostasis is supported by studies of experimental vitamin B_6 and folate deficiencies, showing that oral methionine causes highly elevated blood homocysteine in vitamin B_6 deficiency (31). The fasting hyperhomocysteinemia of folate-deficient rats is attributed to impaired remethylation of homocysteine because of decreased synthesis of methionine and adenosyl methionine (32).

The reactive anhydride, homocysteine thiolactone, is synthesized from methionine in the liver, where it is bound to the lipids of cellular membranes (33). Recent studies have shown that methionyl-tRNA synthase catalyzes synthesis of homocysteine thiolactone from methionine in bacteria by an error-editing reaction (34). This formation of homocysteine thiolactone by error-editing reactions has recently been found to be catalyzed also by isoleucyl- and leucyl-tRNA synthetases (35). Cultured malignant cells accumulate homocysteine thiolactone because of failure of oxidation of the sulfur atom of homocysteine thiolactone to sulfate (36). Malignant cells synthesize homocysteine thiolactone by methionyl-tRNA synthetase (37). The failure of oxidation and overproduction of homocysteine thiolactone in malignant cells are attributed to deficiency of thioretinaco ozonide: a complex of N-homocysteine thiolactonyl retinamide, cobalamin, and ozone (38). The cyclic sulfonium compound S-methyl homocysteine thiolactone is formed from methionine during synthesis of homocysteine thiolactone from methionine (38,39).

In addition to transmethylation of homocysteine by methyl cobalamin, an alternative transmethylation pathway utilizes methyl groups from the methyl donor betaine. Betaine is derived from dietary sources or from oxidation of choline, an important constituent of phosphatidyl choline. Transmethylation of homocysteine by betaine to methionine is catalyzed by betaine homocysteine methyl transferase, an enzyme that is found only in the liver in humans (40). Dietary choline deficiency causes experimental arteriosclerosis in rats (41), a pathological effect that is attributed to hyperhomocysteinemia (5). Recently choline deficiency has been shown to deplete hepatic folate, resulting in hyperhomocysteinemia because of decreased transmethylation of homocysteine by methyl folate (42). Choline deficiency may also result in hyperhomocysteinemia because of decreased transmethylation of homocysteine by the methyl groups of betaine. The methylated sulfur compounds—dimethylthetin, dimethylpropiothetin, and S-methyl methionine—are active in conversion of homocysteine to methionine in rat liver, but the significance of these compounds in preventing human hyperhomocysteinemia has not been studied.

Betaine has been found to lower blood levels of homocysteine in patients with homozygous deficiency of cystathionine synthase that is resistant to pyridoxine therapy (43). However, betaine therapy fails to lower blood homocysteine levels in patients with chronic renal failure maintained on folic acid supplementation (44). The importance of choline, betaine, dimethylthetin, dimethylpropiothetin, S-methyl methionine, and other active methyl donors in the treatment or prevention of human arteriosclerosis has not been explored. These alternative pathways for transmethylation of homocysteine to methionine are illustrated in Fig. 12.2.

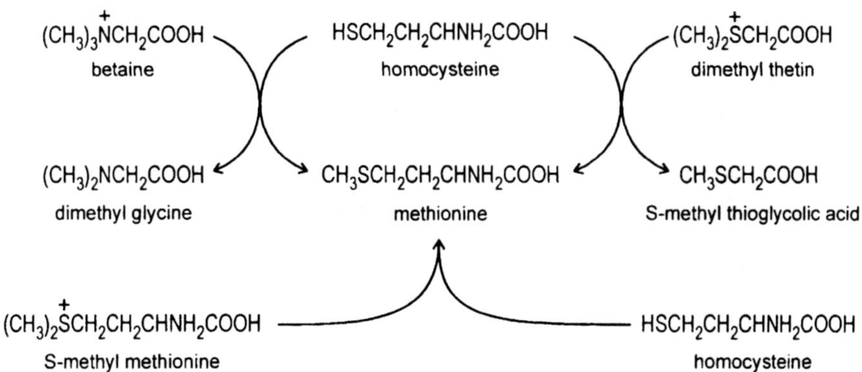

Fig. 12.2. Alternative transmethylation pathways. Methionine is formed by transmethylation reactions that transfer a methyl group from betaine, dimethyl thetin, or S-methyl methionine to the sulfur atom of homocysteine.

Homocysteine, Sulfation, and Macromolecular Conformation

Early studies with cultured cells from the skin of patients with cystathionine synthase deficiency demonstrated that the extracellular proteoglycan matrix is elaborated by these cultured cells in an aggregated conformation (45). Cultured diploid fibroblasts from normal skin elaborate a proteoglycan matrix that is finely fibrillar. Studies of these cultured cells revealed that cystathionine synthase deficiency causes increased binding of inorganic sulfate to the aggregated proteoglycan matrix (46). In experiments with ^{35}S-homocysteine thiolactone a new pathway for sulfate ester synthesis was demonstrated in these cultured cells. Since cystathionine synthesis is blocked, the known pathway (derived from cysteine and inorganic sulfate) could not account for sulfate ester formation in these cells.

The formation of phosphoadenosine phosphosulfate from homocysteic acid (the sulfonic acid derivative of homocysteine) was demonstrated in the liver of normal and scorbutic guinea pigs (47). Homocysteic acid has growth hormone–like effects in hypophysectomized rats treated with thyroxine, increasing cartilage growth and releasing insulinlike growth factor (somatomedin), which increases binding of sulfate to cartilage matrix (48). The formation of inorganic sulfate and phosphoadenosine phosphosulfate from homocysteine thiolactone involves oxidation of the N-homocysteine thiolactonyl retinamide derivative thioretinamide (49) by reactive oxygen radicals (50).

Using an acid hydrolysis method, low-density lipoprotein (LDL) was found to contain increased quantities of homocysteine in persons with hypercholesterolemia (51). LDL contains seven cysteinyl sulfhydryl groups, which are capable of forming cysteine homocysteine disulfides with free homocysteine. In addition, homocysteine reacts with the free amino groups of LDL to form peptide-bound homocysteinyl groups (52). This reaction is known as thiolation because increased numbers of free sulfhydryl groups are introduced into LDL by opening of the five-membered ring of homocysteine thiolactone, resulting in homocysteinylation. Reaction of LDL with increased concentrations of homocysteine thiolactone causes aggregation of LDL (52,53). Studies of this heavily thiolated LDL reveal conversion to a dense form of LDL that is taken up by cultured monocyte-derived macrophages to form foam cells (53). Thiolation of LDL was found to increase internalization of LDL by binding to membrane receptors and by phagocytosis, resulting in increased degradation of LDL and increased cholesterol accumulation within cultured macrophages. However, thiolation of LDL by homocysteine thiolactone did not increase susceptibility of LDL to oxidation by cupric ions *in vitro.*

The overproduction of homocysteine thiolactone by cultured malignant cells (36,37) is attributed to deficiency of thioretinaco ozonide from cellular membranes (38). Increased synthesis of homocysteine thiolactone leads to conversion of cobalamin to thioco and accumulation of oxygen radicals. In addition, homocysteine thiolactone reacts with free amino groups of cellular proteins, forming homocysteinyl groups that are bound by peptide bonds (36). The diffuse abnormalities of cellular membranes and the aggregation of nucleoproteins of chromatin in malignant cells are also attributable to overproduction of homocyteine thiolactone and its reaction with free amino groups of membrane proteins and nucleoproteins.

The free-base form of homocysteine thiolactone, freshly synthesized from the hydrochloride salt, is highly active in causing aggregation of human platelets (54). Injection of homocysteine thiolactone free base into normal mouse tissues causes squamous metaplasia and keratin formation in addition to proliferative effects on stromal and epithelial tissues, necrosis, calcification, and inflammatory reaction (55). The squamous metaplasia and dysplastic changes of gastric mucosa found in a case of homocystinuria, cystathioninuria, and methylmalonic aciduria caused by methyl transferase deficiency are attributable to overproduction of homocysteine thiolactone (6). The inhibition of sulfation in experimental scurvy and the inhibition of sulfomucin formation in retinoid deficiency are attributable to decreased oxidation of thioretinamide (56).

The binding of cations to the negatively charged polyelectrolyte groups of macromolecular biopolymers, including proteins, glycosaminoglycans, and nucleic acids, are known to cause conformational changes in macromolecular structure as well as effects on polarization of water molecules surrounding these polyelectrolyte groups (57). Both the hydrochloride and perchlorate salts of homocysteine thiolactone bind to toluidine blue to cause a metachromatic shift in spectral absorption of light that is attributable to a charge transfer interaction between the dye molecule and the cationic form of homocysteine thiolactone.

As shown in the scheme in Fig. 12.3, homocysteine thiolactone free base forms a stable cationic species by reaction with protons in solution. In addition, the sulfur

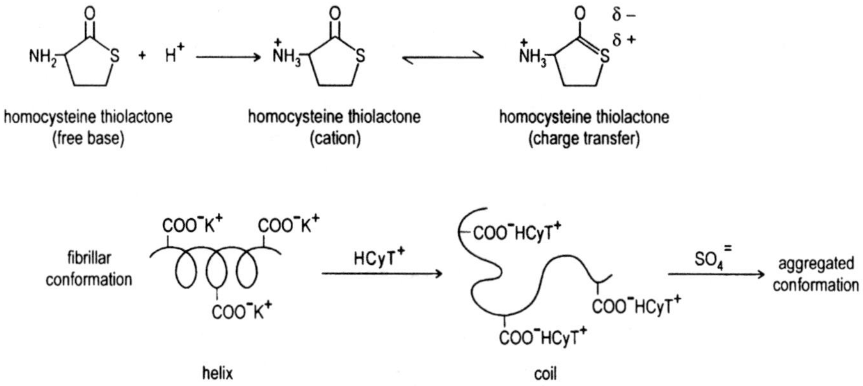

Fig. 12.3. Induction of conformational changes in proteins by homocysteine. The cation of homocysteine thiolactone (HCyT$^+$), which exhibits intramolecular charge transfer characteristics, is adsorbed to acid groups of proteoglycan matrix, low-density lipoprotein, and other macromolecules. Increased binding of sulfate (SO_4^{2-}) produces helix–coil transitions, converting the macromolecule from a fibrillar to an aggregated conformation of decreased solubility.

atom is capable of assuming partial shift of electronic charge to the carbonyl group, producing intramolecular charge transfer. Because of these properties and because of its hydrocarbon ring structure, homocysteine thiolactone free base is soluble in both polar and nonpolar solvents and is uniquely capable of interaction both with the polyanionic groups of macromolecules at physiological pH and with the hydrophobic domains of protein molecules.

The aggregation of low-density lipoprotein and the change in density from loss of core lipids caused by homocysteine thiolactone (53) may be attributed to effects on conformation of apoB protein by interaction with the anionic groups of the protein, causing transitions from helical to random coil, beta sheet, or beta strand conformation, as shown diagrammatically in Figure 12.3. The decreased reactivity with trinitrobenzene sulfonate of low-density lipoprotein treated with high concentrations of homocysteine thiolactone indicates decreased accessibility of free amino groups because of conformational changes and decreased solubility. The increased electrophoretic mobility of heavily thiolated low-density lipoprotein indicates increased surface charge on the particles because of binding of homocysteine thiolactone and anionic solutes to the particle surface. The lipophilic character of the ring of homocysteine thiolactone bound to low-density lipoprotein may protect it from hydrolysis by plasma esterases because of steric restrictions on the active site of the enzyme.

The charge transfer properties of homocysteine thiolactone may contribute to changes in conformation by altering electron distribution along the polypeptide backbone and substituent groups of a wide variety of proteins. A similar effect on proteoglycans may explain the observed conversion from fibrillar to aggregated conformation in cystathionine synthase deficiency cell cultures (45). The scheme in Fig. 12.3 may also explain the decreased solubility of aortic glycoproteins and proteoglycans in a patient with cystathionine synthase deficiency (3). The scheme also explains the increased binding of sulfate anions to proteoglycans observed in cystathionine synthase–deficient cell cultures (46). Although there is little current evidence for a broader effect of homocysteine thiolactone on conformational changes in membrane proteins, keratin polypeptides, and nucleoproteins, future work may implicate the scheme in Fig. 12.3 in a more general context.

Homocysteine, Thioretinaco Ozonide, and Cellular Respiration

The discovery of failure of oxidation of homocysteine thiolactone to sulfate in malignant cell cultures led to the hypothesis that this abnormality of metabolism is caused by loss of a derivative of homocysteine thiolactone from cellular membranes (36). Organic synthesis of antineoplastic derivatives of homocysteine thiolactone and analysis of the biological properties of these model compounds led to several conclusions. The hypothetical derivative is bound to membrane lipids, contains a conjugated double bond system, forms a complex with a transitional metal cation, and contains a carbonyl group adjacent to the amide nitrogen of homocysteine thiolactone. The retinamide of homocysteine thiolactone, thioretinamide, forms a complex with cobalamin, thioretinaco, that is soluble in membrane lipids. These compounds are chemopreventive against chemical carcinogenesis and antineoplastic against transplanted murine carcinomas (49,58).

The abnormality of oxidation of homocysteine in scorbutic guinea pigs (47), the effect of thioretinaco on metabolic activity (58), the observation that oxidized thioethers and oxidized N-acetyl homocysteine thiolactone stimulate ATP synthesis in model systems of oxidative phosphorylation (56,60), and the stimulation of oxidative phosphorylation by ozone (61) suggest participation of the ozonide of thioretinaco in oxidative phosphorylation and cellular respiration (38). In the proposed scheme in Fig. 4 the oxygen–ozone ion cluster, bound to the disulfonium form of thioretinaco, binds ATP from the F_1F_0 complex of mitochondrial membranes. The binding of ATP to the disulfonium active site of thioretinaco ozonide releases ATP, causing proton pumping through the membrane and transport of electrons from electron transport complexes to ubiquinol and the thioretinamide groups of thioretinaco, resulting in reduction of oxygen and stabilization by monodehydroascorbate.

The scheme in Fig. 12.4 is supported by the finding that a synthetic decamethyloctadehydro corrinoid complex of cobalt shunts the respiratory chain of mitochondria, accepting electrons from ubiquinol, donating them to oxygen and

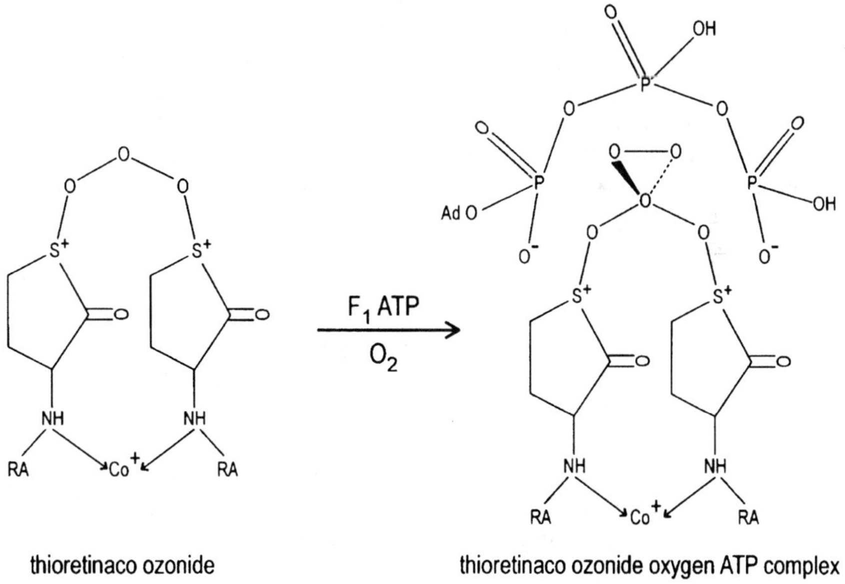

Fig. 12.4. Thioretinaco ozonide in oxidative phosphorylation. Oxygen forms an oxygen–ozone ion cluster with the disulfonium active site of thioretinaco. The stereospecific binding of adenosine triphosphate (ATP) from the F_1F_0 complex of mitochondrial membrane leads to electron transport, reduction of oxygen, and transmembrane proton pumping.

inhibiting the ATPase and ATP synthetase activities of mitochondria (62). Further evidence for this scheme is the finding that ADP ozonide formed from superoxide catalyzes the synthesis of ATP from phosphoric acid (63). An explanation of these results is that the synthetic corrinoid (63) may be able to inhibit the biological activity of thioretinaco ozonide because its structural similarity and lipophilic nature allow competition at the membrane-binding site of thioretinaco ozonide.

The free base of homocysteine thiolactone, freshly synthesized from the hydrochloride salt, is highly toxic when injected into normal mouse tissues; it causes necrosis, calcification, squamous metaplasia, and proliferative changes in stromal and epithelial tissues (55). When applied to the skin surface, homocysteine thiolactone causes epithelial dysplasia and squamous cell carcinoma. The toxic effects on tissues are attributed to the conversion of thioretinaco to thioco and thioretinamide by reaction of homocysteine thiolactone with cobalamin, leading to accumulation of reactive oxygen radicals within tissues because of depletion of the active site for oxidative phosphorylation (56). This reversible alternation among thioretinaco, thioco, and thioretinamide is believed to occur during the normal cell cycle (56). The highly electrophilic character of thioretinaco ozonide characterizes the resting phase of the cell cycle, and the nonelectrophilic character of thioco and its inability to form an electrophilic complex with ozone and oxygen are characteristic of the proliferative phase of the cell cycle. This alternation of thioretinaco, thioco, and thioretinamide with the phases of the cell cycle supports the concept of control of growth by electrophilic substances with inhibitory and stimulatory effects on cell division in normal cells (64).

The involvement of homocysteine in the pathogenesis of arteriosclerosis is based on changes in the oxidative metabolism of vascular cells (29). According to this concept, the homocysteine that is overproduced because of dietary, genetic, senescence, toxic, hormonal, or other etiological factors reacts in its thiolactone form with LDL to form aggregates as illustrated in Fig. 12.3. After these LDL-homocysteine aggregates are taken up by vascular macrophages, the lipid constituents of foam cells are degraded to cholesterol, cholesterol esters, and triglycerides, which are released to form the cholesterol crystals and lipid deposits of advanced plaques.

The homocysteine of LDL-homocysteine aggregates is released in the thiolactone form from foam cells and subsequently reacts with thioretinaco ozonide of vascular wall cells to form thioco, according to current concepts (38). The resulting inhibition of oxidative metabolism leads to accumulation of oxygen radicals, increased deposition of calcium, and formation of oxidized LDL constituents such as oxysterols, aldehydes of fatty acids, and lipid peroxides (65). The increased formation of thioretinamide from thioretinaco ozonide in vascular cells leads to increased formation of proteoglycan sulfates (38). Increased accumulation of oxygen radicals also leads to activation of multiple growth factors and cytokines (66), activation of thrombogenic factors (67), activation of lysosomal elastase, and degeneration of elastic fibers (68), producing hyperplasia of smooth-muscle cells, collagen synthesis, and fibrosis. The final result of these pathophysiological processes is the advanced arteriosclerotic plaque, characterized by intimal damage, thrombogenesis, destruction of elastic interna, deposition of sulfated matrix, hyperplasia of smooth-muscle cells, fibrosis, calcification, and deposition of oxidized lipids and cholesterol crystals (29).

References

1. Mudd, S.H., Skovby, F., Levy, H.L., Pettigrew, K.D., Wilcken, B., Pyertiz, R.E., Andria, G., Boers, G.H.J., Bromberg, I.L., Cerone, R., Fowler, B., Grobe, H., Schmidt, H., and Schweitzer, L. (1985) The Natural History of Homocystinuria Due to Cystathionine Beta Synthase Deficiency, *Am. J. Hum. Genet. 37,* 1–31.

2. Gibson, J.B., Carson, N.A.J., and Neill, D.W. (1964) Pathological Findings in Homocystinuria, *J. Clin. Pathol. 17,* 427–437.

3. Carson, N.A.J., Dent, C.E., Field, C.M.B., and Gaull, G.E. (1965) Homocystinuria. Clinical and Pathological Review of Ten Cases, *J. Pediat. 66,* 565–583.

4. Schimke, R.N., McKusick, V.A., Huang, T., and Pollack, A.D. (1965) Homocystinuria. Studies of 20 Families with 38 Affected Members, *J. Am. Med. Assoc. 193,* 711–719.

5. McCully, K.S. (1969) Vascular Pathology of Homocysteinemia: Implications for the Pathogenesis of Arteriosclerosis, *Am. J. Pathol. 56,* 111–128.

6. McCully, K.S. (1992) Homocystinuria, Arteriosclerosis, Methylmalonic Aciduria, and Methyltransferase Deficiency: A Key Case Revisited, *Nutr. Rev. 50,* 7–12.

7. Kanwar, Y.S., Manaligod, J.R., and Wong, P.W.K. (1976) Morphologic Studies in a Patient with Homocystinuria Due to 5,10-Methylenetetrahydrofolate Reductase Deficiency, *Pediat. Res. 10,* 598–609.

8. McCully, K.S., and Ragsdale, B.D. (1970) Production of Arteriosclerosis by Homocysteinemia, *Am. J. Pathol. 61,* 1–11.

9. Harker, L.A., Ross, R., Slichter, S.J., and Scott, C.R. (1976) Homocystine-Induced Arteriosclerosis. The Role of Endothelial Cell Injury and Platelet Response to Its Genesis, *J. Clin. Invest. 58,* 731–741.

10. McCully, K.S., and Wilson, R.B. (1975) Homocysteine Theory of Arteriosclerosis, *Atherosclerosis 22,* 215–227.

11. McCully, K.S., Olszewski, A.J., and Vezeridis, M.P. (1990) Homocysteine and Lipid Metabolism in Atherogenesis: Effect of the Homocysteine Thiolactonyl Derivatives, Thioretinaco and Thioretinamide, *Atherosclerosis 83,* 197–206.

12. Kuzuya, F., and Yoshimine, N. (1978) Homocysteine Theory of Arteriosclerosis, *(J. Japan Atheroscl. Soc.) 6,* 135–139.

13. Rinehart, J.F., and Greenberg, L.D. (1949) Arteriosclerotic Lesions in Pyridoxine-Deficient Monkeys, *Am. J. Pathol. 25,* 481–491.

14. Smolin, L.A., Crenshaw, T.D., Kurtycz, D., and Benevenga, N.J. (1983) Homocyst(e)ine Accumulation in Pigs Fed Diets Deficient in Vitamin B-6: Relationship to Atherosclerosis, *J. Nutr. 113,* 2122–2133.

15. Wilcken, D.E.L., and Wilcken, B. (1976) The Pathogenesis of Coronary Artery Disease. A Possible Role for Methionine Metabolism, *J. Clin. Invest. 57,* 1079–1082.

16. Boushey, C.J., Beresford, S.A.A., Omenn, G.S., and Motulsky, A.G. (1995) A Quantitative Assessment of Plasma Homocysteine as a Risk Factor for Vascular Disease. Probable Benefits of Increasing Folic Acid Intakes, *J. Am. Med. Assoc. 274,* 1049–1057.

17. Nygard, O., Vollset, S.E., Refsum, H., Stensvold, I., Tverdal, A., Nordrehaug, J.E., and Ueland, P.M. (1995) Total Plasma Homocysteine and Cardiovascular Risk Profile. The Hordaland Homocysteine Study, *J. Am. Med. Assoc. 274,* 1526–1533.

18. Frosst, P., Blom, H.J., Milos, R., Goyette, P., Sheppard, C.A., Matthews, R.G., Boers, G.J.H., den Heijer, M., Kluitjtmans, L.A.J., van den Heuvel, L.P., and Rozen, R. (1995) A Candidate Genetic Risk Factor for Vascular Disease: a Common Mutation in Methylenetetrahydrofolate Reductase, *Nature Genet. 10*, 111–113.

19. Boers, G.H.J., Smals, A.G.H., Trijbels, F.J.M., Fowler, B., Bakkeren, J.A.J.M., Schoonderwaldt, H.C., Kleijer, W.J., and Kloppenborg, P.W.C. (1985) Heterozygosity for Homocystinuria in Premature Peripheral and Cerebral Occlusive Arterial Disease, *New Eng. J. Med. 313*, 709–715.

20. Kozich, V., de Franchis, R., Bowler, B., Boers, G.H.J., Graham, I., and Kraus, J.P. (1995) Hyperhomocysteinemia in Premature Arterial Disease: Examination of Cystathionine Beta Synthase Alleles at the Molecular Level, *Hum. Molec. Genet. 4*, 623–629.

21. Kang, S-S., Wong, P.W.K., and Malinow, M.R. (1992) Hyperhomocysteinemia as a Risk Factor for Occlusive Vascular Disease, *Annu. Rev. Nutr. 12*, 279–298.

22. Selhub, J., Jacques, P.F., Wilson, P.W.F., Rush, D., and Rosenberg, I.H. (1993) Vitamin Status and Intake as Primary Determinants of Homocysteinemia in an Elderly Population, *J. Am. Med. Assoc. 270*, 2693–2698.

23. Selhub, J., Jacques, P.F., Bostom, A.G., D'Agostino, R.B., Wilson, P.W.F., Belanger, A.J., O'Leary, D.H., Wolf, P.A., Schaefer, E.J., and Rosenberg, I.H. (1995) Association between Plasma Homocysteine Concentrations and Extracranial Carotid Artery Stenosis, *New Eng. J. Med. 332*, 286–291.

24. Stampfer, M.J., Malinow, M.R., Willett, W.C., Newcomer, L.M., Upson, B., Ullmann, D., Tishler, P.V., and Hennekens, C.H. (1992) A Prospective Study of Plasma Homocyst(e)ine and Risk of Myocardial Infarction in U.S. Physicians, *J. Am. Med. Assoc. 268*, 877–881.

25. Robinson, K., Mayer, E.L., Miller, D.P., Green, R., van Lente, F., Gupta, A., Kottke-Marchant, K., Savon, S.R., Selhub, J., Nissen, S.E., Kutner, M., Topol, E.J., and Jacobsen, D.W. (1995) Hyperhomocysteinemia and Low Pyridoxal Phosphate. Common and Independent Reversible Risk Factors for Coronary Artery Disease, *Circulation 92*, 2825–2830.

26. Morrison, H.I., Schaubel, D., Desmeules, M., and Wigle, D.T. (1996) Serum Folate and Risk of Fatal Coronary Heart Disease. *J. Am. Med. Assoc. 275*, 1893–1896.

27. Ellis, J.M., and McCully, K.S. (1995) Prevention of Myocardial Infarction by Vitamin B6, *Res. Commun. Molec. Pathol. Pharmacol. 89*, 208–220.

28. McCully, K.S., Homocysteine Theory of Arteriosclerosis: Development and Current Status (1983) in *Atherosclerosis Reviews*, Gotto, A.M., Jr., and Paoletti, R., eds., Raven Press, New York, vol. 11, pp. 157–246.

29. McCully, K.S. (1996) Homocysteine and Vascular Disease, *Nature Med. 2*, 386–389.

30. Selhub, J., and Miller, J.W. (1992) The Pathogenesis of Homocysteinemia: Interruption of the Coordinate Regulation by S-Adenosylmethionine of the Remethylation and Transsulfuration of Homocysteine, *Am. J. Clin. Nutr. 55*, 131–138.

31. Miller, J.W., Nadeau, M.R., Smith, D., and Selhub, J. (1994) Vitamin B-6 Deficiency vs. Folate Deficiency: Comparison of Responses to Methionine Loading in Rats, *Am. J. Clin. Nutr. 59*, 1033–1039.

32. Miller, J.W., Nadeau, M.R., Smith, J. Smith, D., and Selhub, J. (1994) Folate-Deficiency-Induced Homocysteinaemia in Rats: Disruption of S-Adenosylmethionine's Co-Ordinate Regulation of Homocysteine Metabolism, *Biochem. J. 298*, 415–419.

33. Spindel, E., and McCully, K.S. (1974) Conversion of Methionine to Homocysteine Thiolactone in Liver, *Biochem. Biophys. Acta 343*, 687–691.

34. Jakubowski, H. (1990) Proofreading *in vivo:* Editing of Homocysteine by Methionyl-tRNA Synthetase in *Escherichia coli, Proc. Natl. Acad. Sci. USA 87,* 4504–4508.

35. Jakubowski, H. (1995) Proofreading *in vivo:* Editing of Homocysteine by Aminoacyl-tRNA Synthetases in *Escherichia coli, J. Biol. Chem. 270,* 17672–17673.

36. McCully, K.S. (1976) Homocysteine Thiolactone Metabolism in Malignant Cells, *Cancer Res. 36,* 3198–3202.

37. Jakubowski, H., and Goldman, E. (1993) Synthesis of Homocysteine Thiolactone by Methionyl-tRNA Synthetase in Cultured Mammalian Cells, *FEBS Lett. 317,* 237–240.

38. McCully, K.S. (1994) Chemical Pathology of Homocysteine. II. Carcinogenesis and Homocysteine Thiolactone Metabolism, *Ann. Clin. Lab. Sci. 24,* 27–59.

39. Jakubowski, H. (1993) Proofreading and the Evolution of a Methyl Donor Function. Cyclization of Methionine to S-Methyl Homocysteine Thiolactone by *Escherichia coli* Methionyl-tRNA Synthetase, *J. Biol. Chem. 268,* 6549–6553.

40. Wang, J., Dudman, N.P.B., Lynch, J., and Wilcken, D.E.L. (1991) Betaine Homocysteine Methyl Transferase—A New Assay for the Liver Enzyme and Its Absence from Human Skin Fibroblasts and Peripheral Blood Lymphocytes, *Clin. Chem. Acta 204,* 239–250.

41. Hartroft, W.S., Ridout, J.H., Sellers, E.A., and Best, C.H. (1952) Atheromatous Changes in Aorta, Carotid and Coronary Arteries of Choline Deficient Rats, *Proc. Soc. Exp. Biol. Med. 81,* 384–393.

42. Varela-Moreiras, G., Ragel, C., and de Miguelsanz, J. (1995) Choline Deficiency and Methotrexate Treatment Induces Marked but Reversible Changes in Hepatic Folate Concentrations, Serum Homocysteine and DNA Methylation Rates in Rats, *J. Am. Coll. Nutr. 14,* 480–485.

43. Wilcken, D.E.L., Wilcken, B., Dudman, N.P.B., and Tyrrell, P.A. (1983) Homocystinuria —The Effects of Betaine in the Treatment of Patients Not Responsive to Pyridoxine, *New Eng. J. Med. 309,* 448–453.

44. Bostom, A.G., Shemin, D., Nadeau, M., Shih, V., Stabler, S.P., Allen, R.H., and Selhub, J. (1995) Short Term Betaine Therapy Fails to Lower Elevated Fasting Total Plasma Homocysteine Concentrations in Hemodialysis Patients Maintained on Chronic Folic Acid Supplementation, *Atherosclerosis 113,* 129–132.

45. McCully, K.S. (1970) Importance of Homocysteine-Induced Abnormalities of Proteoglycan Structure in Arteriosclerosis, *Am. J. Pathol. 59,* 181–193.

46. McCully, K.S. (1972) Macromolecular Basis for Homocysteine-Induced Changes in Proteoglycan Structure in Growth and Arteriosclerosis, *Am. J. Pathol. 66,* 83–95.

47. McCully, K.S. (1971) Homocysteine Metabolism in Scurvy, Growth and Arteriosclerosis, *Nature 231,* 391–392.

48. Clopath P., Smith, V.C., and McCully, K.S. (1976) Growth Promotion by Homocysteic Acid, *Science 192,* 372–374.

49. McCully, K.S., and Vezeridis, M.P. (1987) Chemopreventive and Antineoplastic Activity of N-Homocysteine Thiolactonyl Retinamide, *Carcinogenesis 8,* 1559–1562.

50. McCully, K.S. (1993) Chemical Pathology of Homocysteine. I. Atherogenesis, *Ann. Clin. Lab. Sci. 24,* 477–493.

51. Olszewski, A.J., and McCully, K.S. (1991) Homocysteine Content of Lipoproteins in Hypercholesterolemia, *Atherosclerosis 88,* 61–68.

52. Vidal, M., Sainte-Marie, J., Philippot, J., and Bienvenue, A. (1986) Thiolation of Low Density Lipoproteins and Their Interaction with L_2C Leukemic Lymphocytes, *Biochimie 68,* 723–730.

53. Naruszewicz, M, Mirkiewicz, E., Olszewski, A.J. and McCully, K.S. (1994) Thiolation of Low-Density Lipoprotein by Homocysteine Thiolactone Causes Increased Aggregation and Altered Interaction with Cultured Macrophages, *Nutr. Metab. Cardiovas. Dis.* *4*, 70–77.

54. McCully, K.S., and Carvalho, A.C.A. (1987) Homocysteine Thiolactone, N-Homocysteine Thiolactonyl Retinamide, and Platelet Aggregation, *Res. Commun. Chem. Pathol. Pharmacol. 56*, 349–360.

55. McCully, K.S., and Vezeridis, M.P. (1989) Histopathological Effects of Homocysteine Thiolactone on Epithelial and Stromal Tissues, *Exp. Molec. Pathol. 51*, 159–170.

56. McCully, K.S. (1994) Chemical Pathology of Homocysteine. III. Cellular Function and Aging, *Ann. Clin. Lab. Sci. 24*, 134–152.

57. Wiggins, P.M. (1990) Role of Water in Some Biological Processes, *Microbiol. Rev. 54*, 432–449.

58. McCully, K.S., and Vezeridis, M.P. (1989) Chemopreventive Effect of N-Homocysteine Thiolactonyl Retinamido Cobalamin on Carcinogensis by Ethyl Carbamate in Mice, *Proc. Soc. Exp. Biol. Med. 191*, 346–351.

59. Lambeth, D.O., and Lardy, H.A. (1969) The Oxidation of Thioethers by Bromine: A Model System for Oxidative Phosphorylation, *Biochemistry 8*, 3395–3402.

60. Wieland, T., and Bauerlein, E. (1967) N-acetyl Homocysteine Thiolactone als Vermitter einer Oxydativen Synthese von Adenosindiphosphat und Adenosintriphosphat und Orthophosphat, *Chem. Ber. 100*, 3869–3876.

61. Mustafa, M.G., DeLuca, A.J., York, G.K., Arth, C., and Cross, C.E. (1973) Ozone Interaction with Rodent Lung. II. Effects on Oxygen Consumption of Mitochondria, *J. Lab. Clin. Med. 82*, 357–365.

62. Kiseleva, L.L., Novodarova, G.N., Vol'pin, M.E., and Vinogradov, A.D. (1982) Influence of a Cobalt Dehydrocorrin Complex on Mitochondria, *Biokhimiya 47*, 1877–1882.

63. Lippman, R.D. (1982) A New Method That Investigates Superoxide versus Respiration *in vitro* Using Bioluminescence and Sepharose-Bound Adenosine Derivatives, *J. Biochem. Biophys. Meth. 6*, 81–87.

64. Szent-Gyorgi, A. (1965) Cell Division and Cancer, *Science 149*, 34–37.

65. Olszewski, A.J., and McCully, K.S. (1993) Homocysteine Metabolism and the Oxidative Modification of Proteins and Lipids, *Free Rad. Biol. Med. 14*, 683–693.

66. Ross. R. (1993) The Pathogenesis of Atherosclerosis: A Perspective for the 1990s, *Nature 362*, 801–809.

67. Rees, M.M., and Rodgers, G.M. (1993) Homocysteinemia: Association of a Metabolic Disorder with Vascular Disease and Thrombosis, *Thromb. Res. 71*, 337–359.

68. Rolland, P.H., Friggi, A., Barlatier, A., Piquet, P., Latrille, V., Faye, N.M., Guillon, J., Charpiot, P., Bodard, H., Ghiringhelli, O., Calef, R., Luccioni, R., and Garcon, D. (1995) Hyperhomocysteinemia-Induced Vascular Damage in the Minipig. Captopril-Hydrochlorothiazide Combination Prevents Elastic Alterations, *Circulation 91*, 1161–1174.

Chapter 13

Choline and Choline Esters as Required Nutrients During Pregnancy and Lactation

Steven H. Zeisel

Department of Nutrition, School of Public Health and School of Medicine, The University of North Carolina at Chapel Hill, Chapel Hill, NC 27599-7400

Introduction

Of all the different dietary components available to the human body, choline is one of the most important. Not only does choline support the structural integrity and signaling functions of cell membranes (1); it also directly affects cholinergic neurotransmission, lipid transport, and metabolism (1).

Phospholipids such as phosphatidylcholine and sphingomyelin, which contain most of the body's choline, play important roles. Phosphatidylcholine is the predominant phospholipid in most mammalian membranes (>50%); disaturated phosphatidylcholine is the major active component of surfactant in the lungs (2), a deficiency of which can lead to respiratory distress syndrome in premature infants. Other choline metabolites important to the body include platelet-activating factor, acetylcholine, choline plasmalogens, lysophosphatidylcholine, phosphocholine, glycerophosphocholine, and betaine. Finally, choline is important as the major source of methyl groups in the diet (1). Several comprehensive reviews of the metabolism and functions of choline (1,3) discuss these functions in great detail. For the purposes of this paper we can simply state that choline is essential to a cell's ability to function normally.

The Nutritional Importance of Choline

When healthy male subjects are deprived of dietary choline, plasma concentrations of choline and phosphatidylcholine drop, and the men develop symptoms of incipient liver dysfunction (4). Likewise, when malnourished patients are treated with total parenteral nutrition (TPN) solutions—which contain little or no choline—their choline stores become depleted, and fatty liver syndrome and hepatic dysfunction set in. When choline (in the form of lecithin) is reintroduced to the deficient patient, the hepatic steatosis reverses (5).

Choline's role as a methyl donor may play a significant role in the development of tissues early in life. Choline, methionine, and methyl folate are closely interrelated, with their pathways intersecting where homocysteine is converted into methionine. In one pathway, betaine:homocysteine methyltransferase catalyzes the methylation of homocysteine using betaine as the methyl donor (6) A separate pathway uses a methyl group derived *de novo* from the 1-carbon folate pool (6) to regenerate methionine from 5-methyltetrahydrofolate:homocysteine methyltransferase. Should choline deficiency perturb the metabolism of one of the methyl donors, these two pathways mingle, resulting in compensatory changes in the other methyl donors (7–9). Consider, for example, that rats fed a choline-deficient diet show diminished tissue concentrations of methionine and S-adenosylmethionine (8) and a decrease in total folate (9), whereas rats treated with methotrexate (a folate antagonist) show diminished pools of choline metabolites in liver (10). If inadequate choline can complicate folate and homocysteine metabolism and thus cause folate deficiency, the result in humans—especially pregnant humans—can be serious. Multiple studies have demonstrated that humans with diminished folate status are much more likely to have babies with neural tube defects (11,12). In studies with mice, folate deficiency appeared to increase rates of exencephaly (13).

Choline is not hard to get. Many foods in the human diet contain choline, sphingomyelin, and phosphatidylcholine naturally; other foods have choline added during food processing (especially when preparing infant formula (14)). While no information yet exists about the phosphocholine or glycerophosphocholine content in foods, it is likely that these components occur in the human diet, too.

Increased Availability of Choline to Tissues During and Following Pregnancy

Choline availability is especially important during and immediately after pregnancy for two reasons: First, a neonate requires choline for proper organ growth and for organ membrane biosynthesis (1,15). Second, choline appears to affect brain development during the neonatal period, further increasing its importance during the first weeks of life. When rat pups received choline supplements (some *in utero,* others during the second week after birth), their brain function changed, resulting in lifelong memory enhancement (16–18).

The human body distributes choline to tissues with great efficiency, delivering choline when and where it is needed most. Evidently, choline is most important perinatally, because plasma or serum choline concentrations are highest *in utero* and then decline progressively during the first weeks after birth (19), measuring six- to sevenfold higher in the fetus and neonate than in the adult (20, 21). We can presume that the high levels of choline circulating in the neonate ensure choline's availability to the developing baby.

While choline levels are highest during the perinatal period, the baby's changing requirements for and metabolism of choline cause fluctuation in its availability. Studies show that neonatal rat brain extracts choline from blood much better than adult brain does (22–25); increased serum choline in the newborn rat is associated with twofold higher choline concentration in neonatal brain than is present later in life. Furthermore, supplementing choline during the perinatal period further increases blood and brain choline metabolite concentrations (26).

Pregnant Animals Deplete Their Choline Reserves

While fetal tissues contain significant amounts of choline, choline concentrations measured in maternal blood are relatively low (12 µM) (19). As with most nutrients, the fetus derives choline from maternal blood. A transport system in the maternal placenta pumps the choline into the fetus against a concentration gradient (27–31). The placenta is one of the few non-nervous tissues that stores large amounts of choline as acetylcholine (32), suggesting that the acetylcholine in the placenta may be a special reserve storage pool that ensures delivery of choline to the fetus.

Transporting choline from the mother to the fetus depletes the mother's stores of choline; liver choline concentration falls from a mean of 130 µM in adult nonpregnant rats to 38 µM in late pregnancy (33,34). Since liver phosphocholine is the most reliable marker for changes in choline status, a recent study comparing liver phosphocholine in pregnant female rats to levels in male and nonmated female rats is of particular interest (35). Pregnant rats eating a standard rat diet (AIN-76A diet) for 6 days (days 12–18 gestation), were compared to nonmated female rats eating the same diets (Fig. 13.1). The nonmated female rats on the control diet had higher concentrations of hepatic choline metabolites than either the male rats (choline, 98% higher; betaine, 96% higher; and phosphocholine, 55% higher; data not shown in Fig. 13.1), the pregnant rats, or the lactating rats.

Liver phosphocholine levels in male adult rats were the most sensitive to modest dietary choline deficiency, decreasing to 10–20% of control values after only a short time on an AIN-76A diet without added choline (10). The nonmated females showed only a modest decrease of phosphocholine in liver on the choline-deficient diet, compared with those that ate the control diet (33% decrease). In the pregnant rats, a choline-deficient diet resulted in a more significant drop of hepatic phosphocholine (83% decrease) than was measured in the nonmated females (35). While this study shows that nonmated female rats tolerate choline deficiency better than male rats, it also shows that, once pregnant, the females lose this tolerance and become more vulnerable to choline deficiency than the males are. A decreased demand for methylation and an enhanced capacity to form the choline moiety *de novo* may explain the relative resistance of nonmated females to choline deficiency. Creatinine formation is a major sink for methyl groups; therefore a male body, with its greater muscle mass, may demand more methyl groups than the female body (36). As a result, females may use less choline (in the form of betaine) as a methyl donor.

Choline is synthesized *de novo* through only one pathway in the mammal. Catalyzed by phosphatidylethanolamine N-methyltransferase activity, this pathway forms phosphatidylcholine by using methyl groups from S-adenosylmethionine and phosphatidylethanolamine (37). Although most phosphatidylethanolamine N-methyltransferase activity occurs in the liver (38), the activity also occurs in brain (39) and other tissues (40). In brain tissue the phosphatidylethanolamine N-methyltransferase pathway is located in the nerve endings (41).

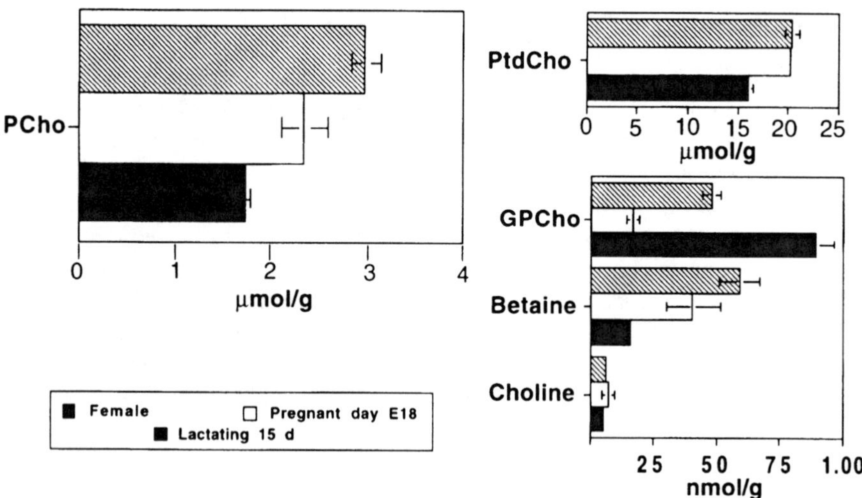

Fig. 13.1. Pregnancy and lactation diminish concentrations of choline and its metabolites in rat liver. Pregnant and nonmated female rats were fed a standard AIN-76A diet for 6 days (starting the evening of day 12 of gestation in the pregnant rats). Lactating and non-mated female rats were fed a standard AIN-76A diet for 25 days (starting the evening of day 12 of gestation in the pregnant rats). Animals were killed and liver collected and analyzed for choline metabolites as described in methods. PtdCho = phosphatidylcholine; PCho = phosphorylcholine; GPCho = glycerophosphorylcholine. Data are expressed as mean ± SEM for at least 6 rats per point. (*Source:* Modified from Ref. 35, with permission.)

Phosphatidylethanolamine N-methyltransferase activity in certain tissues appears to be influenced by sex hormones (42). For example, females have greater phosphatidylethanolamine N-methyltransferase activity in liver than males do (38, 43,44); estimates of increased activity range from 10 (44) to 50% (38). Along these same lines, the incorporation rate of methyls from methionine into phosphatidylcholine is much greater in young women than in postmenopausal women (45), again suggesting a hormonal influence. Other examples of hormonal links to phosphatidylethanolamine N-methyltransferase activity include studies in which 17 β-estradiol significantly increased phosphatidylethanolamine N-methyltransferase activity in pituitary cells, whereas 17 α-estradiol (an inactive stereoisomer of 17 β-estradiol) had no effect (42,46). Another experiment showed that estrogen increased phosphatidylethanolamine N-methyltransferase activity in estradiol-treated, castrated male rats but not in similarly treated, noncastrated rats—suggesting that testosterone may interact with estradiol (47).

The depletion of choline stores evident in pregnant rats indicates that demand for choline exceeds the capacity of the combination of dietary intake and *de novo* synthesis during pregnancy.

Lactation Exacerbates the Choline Depletion That Starts in Pregnancy

Most of the choline and choline esters in human and rat milk (approximately 2 mmol/L) is pulled from maternal plasma (48–50). As a result, the mother experiences an appreciable drain on her choline stores, making her even more vulnerable to the effects of choline deficiency she was at risk for during pregnancy. Nonmated female rats eating a defined control diet for 25 days (gestation day 12–postpartum day 15) had higher hepatic choline metabolite concentrations than did lactating rats on an identical diet (phosphocholine, 49% higher; phosphatidylcholine, 37% higher; and betaine, 273% higher) (35) (Fig. 13.1). On the other hand, eating a choline-deficient diet for 25 days (gestation day 12–postpartum day 15) made lactating rats more sensitive to choline deficiency, with levels of liver phosphocholine decreasing 88%, compared to a 12% decrease observed in nonmated females (35).

Milk as a Source of Choline

A lactating female's vulnerability to choline deficiency can be linked to her milk production. Mother's milk is an excellent source of unesterified choline, phosphocholine, and glycerophosphocholine (48, 49) (Fig. 13.2), with concentrations being highest immediately following parturition (50). However, exactly how glycerophosphocholine makes its way into the milk is still being determined. It may be derived from maternal plasma, as label from plasma appears in glycerophosphocholine in milk (26); or it is also possible that maternal organs—including mammary glands (mammary epithelial cells are known to synthesize and secrete glycerophosphocholine)—synthesize the glycerophosphocholine. Glycerophosphocholine is formed from phosphatidylcholine by the action of phospholipases A_1 and A_2 or by glycerophosphocholine diesterase (51). But in milk, phosphatidylcholine is not hydrolyzed into glycerophosphocholine (50).

We know that milk fat globule membranes contain the phospholipids sphingomyelin and phosphatidylcholine (48, 50); and we know that most cells contain large amounts of phosphocholine (52). We also know that mammary cells phosphorylate choline to create phosphocholine (49) and that phosphocholine can be converted into phosphatidylcholine (53) and then form glycerophosphocholine (49). The glycerophosphocholine concentration of the mammary cell is approximately 10% of the concentration present in milk, suggesting that this choline-compound is transported against a concentration gradient.

Human milk is not a static food; its composition changes with time postnatally. Colostrum and transitional milk contain approximately 2 mmol/L choline moiety (500 µmol/L free choline, 400 µmol/L choline in phospholipids (50) and 800 µmol/L choline as glycerophosphocholine and phosphocholine), whereas total choline intake in the adult human is >70–100 µmol kg^{-1} d^{-1} (4,54). The choline intake of a newborn human infant who drank 150 mL kg^{-1} d^{-1} of milk would be

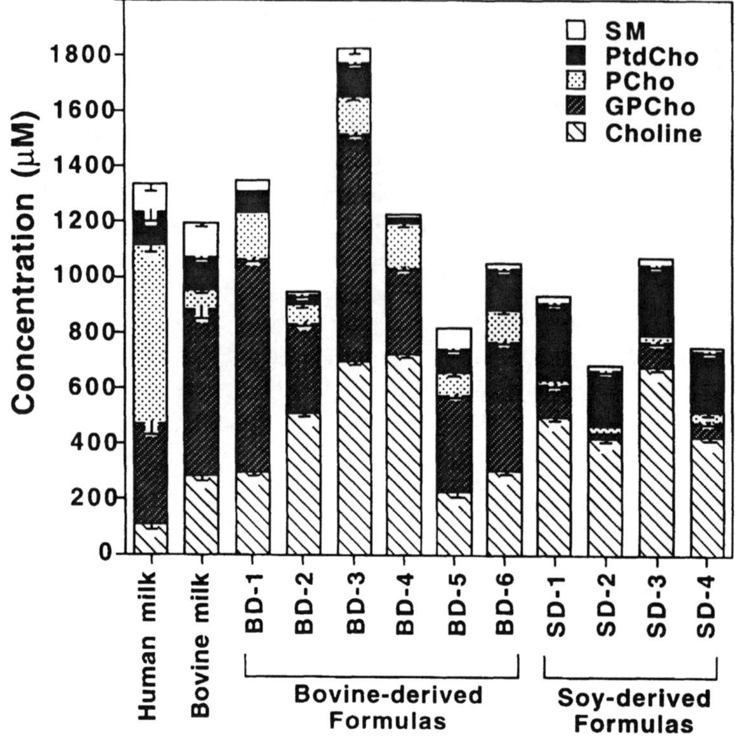

Fig. 13.2. Choline and choline ester content of human milk, bovine milk, and infant formulas. Human and bovine milks and infant formulas were analyzed for choline content using GC/mass spectrometry. Data are expressed as mean concentration (μmol/L) in human milk (n = 33/point), bovine milk (n = 3/point), and commercial powdered infant formulas (n = 3/point), either bovine-derived (BD) or soy-derived (SD). *Abbreviations:* GPCho, glycerophosphocholine; PCho, phosphocholine; PtdCho, phosphatidylcholine; SM, sphingomyelin. Variability of data is indicated as SEM within the stacked bar for the data; when error bars are not shown, they were smaller than could be indicated by an error bar. (*Source:* Ref. 48, with permission.)

approximately 200–250 μmol kg^{-1} d^{-1}—two to three times that ingested by the adult human.

Supplemental choline in the rat is concentrated into the dam's milk (55). When lactating rat dams consume either a choline-deficient or choline-supplemented diet, significant changes in the milk's phosphocholine concentration result (48). As mentioned earlier, dietary choline is just as important to neonates as it is to adults. Rat pups denied access to milk have lower serum choline concentrations than do their fed litter mates (20), suggesting that dietary intake of choline contributes to the high serum choline concentrations in the newborn. Lactating humans consuming a low-choline diet had lower milk choline concentrations than those eating adequate amounts of choline (56). Interestingly, while milk phosphocholine concentration was reduced by 50% on the choline deficient diet in the rat, other choline compounds remain unchanged (48). Conversely, milk phosphocholine concentrations increase when rats consume a choline-supplemented diet, while other choline compounds are unchanged (48). This dietary variation causes a fourfold change in milk phosphocholine content between the choline-deficient and choline-supplemented diets.

Where does all of this choline in milk come from? Mammary epithelial cells can transport choline from maternal blood via two ways (57). One method is saturable with Michaelis-Menten kinetics; the other method is nonsaturable and linear. As mentioned previously, research has shown that mammary epithelial cells can synthesize choline *de novo* (40) via phosphatidylethanolamine N-methyltransferase activity.

Human milk is the gold standard from which we calculate infants' nutrient requirements and from which infant formulas are designed (58–60). Commercially made infant formulas as well as bovine milk contain choline and choline-containing compounds (48), but human milk has significantly higher phosphocholine (718 μmol/L) concentration than do either bovine milk or infant formulas. On the other hand, bovine milk and bovine-derived infant formulas have the same or higher glycerophosphocholine concentration (400–800 μmol/L) than does human milk (415 μmol/L), and soy-based infant formulas contain lower glycerophosphocholine concentrations (115 μmol/L or less) than human milk. Concentrations of phosphatidylcholine and sphingomyelin in human milk do not differ greatly from those in bovine milk and bovine-derived infant formulas (200 μmol/L) (48). Soy-derived infant formulas, on the other hand, have more phosphatidylcholine than do either human milk or bovine-derived formulas but contain less sphingomyelin than human milk. Unesterified choline concentration in mature human milk is 30–80% lower than in either bovine milk or the infant formulas. Mature human milk has significantly lower free choline than do colostrum and transitional human milk (50).

The bioavailability of water-soluble, choline-derived compounds (choline, phosphocholine, and glycerophosphocholine) differs noticeably from that of the lipid-soluble compounds (phosphatidylcholine and sphingomyelin) that are present in milk (61). For example, choline is first absorbed by the intestinal mucosa and then by the liver (61), where it is transported in the blood to other tissues, such as brain. Liver tissue metabolizes phosphatidylcholine-derived label differently from other choline esters, with most of the choline remaining (and perhaps being incorporated) in the liver as phosphatidylcholine. Once absorbed by the liver, a portion of the phosphatidylcholine is secreted as plasma lipoprotein (1). The glycerophosphocholine ingested in milk is metabolized differently in the liver than either the choline or the phosphocholine.

It is worth considering, then, that formulas and milks with different dietary compositions may deliver choline in different amounts and different forms, potentially upsetting the balance between choline's use as a methyl donor (*via* betaine), an acetylcholine precursor (*via* choline), or or phospholipid precursor (*via* phosphocholine and phosphatidylcholine). While the data obtained from the rat pup model cannot be directly extrapolated to the human infant, data indicate that variations in the bioavailability and utilization of choline, phosphocholine, glycerophosphocholine, and phosphatidylcholine in milk should be considered when milk substitutes are developed. In the design of infant formulas, careful use of human milk as a model will provide a safe and effective system of delivering choline to the newborns.

Summary

Pregnancy and lactation are periods when choline deficiency is most dangerous to mother and child. Ironically, pregnancy and lactation are also the periods when choline deficiency is most likely. The developing fetus and newborn require significant amounts of choline for normal development of their internal organs and brain, often drawing that choline from—and thus depleting—maternal reserves *in utero* and when nursing. Choline deficiency in the mother can result in liver dysfunction and potential disturbance of methyl group formation; choline deficiency in the baby can retard organ development and brain/memory function. These observations are important for the obstetrician and pediatrician as they consider the ideal dietary intake for mothers and their children.

Acknowledgments

Some of the work described in this review was supported by a grant from the National Institutes of Health (AG09525). I thank Lisa Canada and Janet Wagner for their help in editing this manuscript, and I thank my students and collaborators for performing much of the work that I describe.

References

1. Zeisel, S.H., and Blusztajn, J.K. (1994) Choline and Human Nutrition, *Ann. Rev. Nutr. 14*, 269–296.
2. Brown, E.S. (1964) Isolation and Assay of Dipalmitoyl Lecithin in Lung Extracts, *Am. J. Physiol. 207*, 402–406.
3. Zeisel, S.H. (1993) in *Modern Nutrition in Health and Disease,* Shils, M.E., Olson, J.A., and Shike, M., eds., 8th edn., Lea & Febiger, Philadelphia, pp. 449–458.
4. Zeisel, S.H., Da Costa, K.-A., Franklin, P.D., Alexander, E.A., Lamont, J.T., Sheard, N.F., and Beiser, A. (1991) Choline, an Essential Nutrient for Humans, *FASEB J. 5*, 2093–2098.
5. Buchman, A.L., Dubin, M., Jenden, D., Moukarzel, A., Roch, M.H., Rice, K., Gornbein, J., Ament, M.E., and Eckhert, C.D. (1992) Lecithin Increases Plasma Free Choline and Decreases Hepatic Steatosis in Long-Term Total Parenteral Nutrition Patients, *Gastroenterol. 102*, 1363–1370.
6. Finkelstein, J.D., Martin, J.J., Harris B.J., and Kyle, W.E. (1983) Regulation of Hepatic Betaine-Homocysteine Methyltransferase by Dietary Betaine, *J. Nutr. 113*, 519–521.
7. Varela-Moreiras, G., Selhub, J., da Costa. K., and Zeisel, S.H. (1992) Effect of Chronic Choline Deficiency in Rats on Liver Folate Content and Distribution, *J. Nutr. Biochem. 3*, 519–522.

8. Zeisel, S.H., Zola, T., da Costa, K., and Pomfret, E.A. (1989) Effect of Choline Deficiency on S-Adenosylmethionine and Methionine Concentrations in Rat Liver, *Biochem. J. 259*, 725–729.

9. Selhub, J., Seyoum, E., Pomfret, E.A., and Zeisel, S.H. (1991) Effects of Choline Deficiency and Methotrexate Treatment upon Liver Folate Content and Distribution, *Cancer Res. 51*, 16–21.

10. Pomfret, E.A., da Costa, K., and Zeisel, S.H. (1990) Effects of Choline Deficiency and Methotrexate Treatment upon Rat Liver, *J. Nutr. Biochem. 1*, 533–541.

11. Rush, D. (1994) Periconceptional Folate and Neural Tube Defect, *Am. J. Clin. Nutr. 59*, 511S–515S.

12. Milunsky, A., Jick, H., Jick, S.S., Bruell, C.L., MacLaughlin, D.S., Rothman, K.J., and Willett, W. (1989) Multivitamin/Folic Acid Supplementation in Early Pregnancy Reduces the Prevalence of Neural Tube Defects, *J. Am. Med. Assoc. 262*, 2847–2852.

13. Trotz, M., Wegner, C.H.R., and Nau, H. (1987) Valproic Acid Induced Neural Tube Defects: Reproduction by Folinic Acid in the Mouse, *Life Sci. 41*, 103–110.

14. FASEB Life Sciences Research Office (1975) *Evaluation of the Health Aspects of Choline Chloride and Choline Bitartrate as Food Ingredients: Report # PB-223 845/9*, Bureau of Foods, Food and Drug Administration, Department of Health, Education, and Welfare, Washington, D.C.

15. Zeisel, S.H. (1992) Choline: An Important Nutrient in Brain Development, Liver Function and Carcinogenesis, *J. Am. Coll. Nutr. 11*, 473–481.

16. Meck, W.H., Smith, R.A., and Williams, C.L. (1989) Organizational Changes in Cholinergic Activity and Enhanced Visuospatial Memory as a Function of Choline Administered Prenatally or Postnatally or Both, *Behav. Neurosci. 103*, 1234–1241.

17. Meck, W.H., Smith, R.A., and Williams, C.L. (1988) Pre- and Postnatal Choline Supplementation Produces Long-Term Facilitation of Spatial Memory, *Dev. Psychobiol. 21*, 339–353.

18. Loy, R., Heyer, D., Williams, C.L., and Meck, W.H. (1991) Choline-Induced Spatial Memory Facilitation Correlates with Altered Distribution and Morphology of Septal Neurons, *Adv. Exp. Med. Biol. 295*, 373–382.

19. McMahon, K.E., and Farrell, P.M. (1985) Measurement of Free Choline Concentrations in Maternal and Neonatal Blood by Micropyrolysis Gas Chromatography, *Clin. Chem. Acta 149*, 1–12.

20. Zeisel, S.H., and Wurtman, R.J. (1981) Developmental Changes in Rat Blood Choline Concentration, *Biochem. J. 198*, 565–570.

21. Zeisel, S.H., Epstein, M.F., and Wurtman, R.J. (1980) Elevated Choline Concentration in Neonatal Plasma, *Life Sci. 26*, 1827–1831.

22. Cornford, E.M., Braun, L.D., and Oldendorf, W.H. (1982) Developmental Modulations of Blood-Brain Barrier Permeability as an Indicator of Changing Nutritional Requirements in the Brain, *Pediatr. Res. 16*, 324–328.

23. Cornford, E.M., Braun L.D., and Oldendorf, W.H. (1978) Carrier Mediated Blood-Brain Barrier Transport of Choline and Certain Choline Analogs, *J. Neurochem. 30*, 299–308.

24. Braun, L.D., Cornford, E.M., and Oldendorf, W.H. (1980) Newborn Rabbit Blood-Brain Barrier is Selectively Permeable and Differs Substantially from the Adult, *J. Neurochem. 34*, 147–152.

25. Cornford, E.M., and Cornford, M.E. (1986) Nutrient Transport and the Blood-Brain Barrier in Developing Animals, *Fed. Proc. 45*, 2065–2072.

26. Garner, S.C., Mar, M.-H., and Zeisel, S.H. (1995) Choline Distribution and Metabolism in Pregnant Rats and Fetuses Are Influenced by the Choline Content of the Maternal Diet, *J. Nutr. 125*, 2851–2858.

27. Yudilevich, D.L., and Sweiry, J.H. (1985) Membrane Carriers and Receptors at Maternal and Fetal Sides of the Placenta by Single Circulation Paired-Tracer Dilution: Evidence for a Choline Transport System, *Contrib. Gynecol. Obstet. 13*, 158–161.

28. Sweiry, J.H., and Yudilevich, D.L. (1985) Characterization of Choline Transport at Maternal and Fetal Interfaces of the Perfused Guinea-Pig Placenta, *J. Physiol. 366*, 251–266.

29. Sweiry, J.H., Page, K.R., Dacke, C.G., Abramovich, D.R., and Yudilevich, D.L. (1986) Evidence of Saturable Uptake Mechanisms at Maternal and Fetal Sides of the Perfused Human Placenta by Rapid Paired-Tracer Dilution: Studies with Calcium and Choline, *J. Dev. Physiol. 8*, 435–445.

30. Welsch, F., Wenger, W.C., and Stedman D.B. (1981) Choline Metabolism in Placenta: Evidence for the Biosynthesis of Phosphatidylcholine in Microsomes Via the Methylation Pathway, *Placenta 2*, 211–221.

31. Welsch, F. (1978) Choline Metabolism in Human Term Placenta—Studies on De Novo Synthesis and the Effects of Some Drugs on the Metabolic Fate of [N-methyl ^{3}H]Choline, *Biochem. Pharmacol. 27*, 1251–1257.

32. Leventer, S.M., and Rowell, P.P. (1984) Investigation of the Rate-Limiting Step in the Synthesis of Acetylcholine by the Human Placenta, *Placenta 5*, 261–270.

33. Gwee, M.C., and Sim, M.K. (1979) Changes in the Concentration of Free Choline and Cephalin-N-methyltransferase Activity of the Rat Maternal and Foetal Liver and Placenta During Gestation and of the Maternal and Neonatal Liver in the Early Postpartum Period, *Clin. Exp. Pharmacol. Physiol. 6*, 259–265.

34. Gwee, M.C., and Sim, M.K. (1978) Free Choline Concentration and Cephalin-N-methyltransferase Activity in the Maternal and Foetal Liver and Placenta of Pregnant Rats, *Clin. Exp. Pharmacol. Physiol. 5*, 649–653.

35. Zeisel, S.H., Mar, M.-H., Zhou, Z.-W., and da Costa, K.-A. (1995) Pregnancy and Lactation Are Associated with Diminished Concentrations of Choline and Its Metabolites in Rat Liver, *J. Nutr. 125*, 3049–3054.

36. Mudd, S.H., and Poole, J.R. (1975) Labile Methyl Balances for Normal Humans on Various Dietary Regimens, *Metab. Clin. Exp. 24*, 721–735.

37. Bremer, J., and Greenberg, D. (1961) Methyl Transferring Enzyme System of Microsomes in the Biosynthesis of Lecithin (Phosphatidylcholine), *Biochim. Biophys. Acta 46*, 205–216.

38. Bjornstad, P., and Bremer, J. (1966) In Vivo Studies on Pathways for the Biosynthesis of Lecithin in the Rat, *J. Lipid Res. 7*, 38–45.

39. Blusztajn, J.K., Zeisel, S.H., and Wurtman, R.J. (1979) Synthesis of Lecithin (Phosphatidylcholine) from Phosphatidylethanolamine in Bovine Brain, *Brain Res. 179*, 319–327.

40. Yang, E.K., Blusztajn, J.K., Pomfret, E.A., and Zeisel, S.H. (1988) Rat and Human Mammary Tissue Can Synthesize Choline Moiety Via the Methylation of Phosphatidylethanolamine, *Biochem. J. 256*, 821–828.

41. Blusztajn, J.K., Zeisel, S.H., and Wurtman, R.J. (1981) Phospholipid Methylation and Cholinergic Neurons in *Biochemistry of S-Adenosylmethionine and Related Compounds*, Wurtman, R.J., ed., MacMillan Press Ltd., Lake of the Ozarks, Missouri, pp. 155–164.

42. Drouva, S.V., LaPlante, E., Leblanc, P., Bechet J.J., Clauser, H., and Kordon, C. (1986) Estradiol Activates Methylating Enzyme(s) Involved in the Conversion of Phosphatidylethanolamine to Phosphatidylcholine in Rat Pituitary Membranes, *Endocrinol. 119*, 2611–2622.

43. Arvidson, G.A. (1968) Biosynthesis of Phosphatidylcholines in Rat Liver, *Europ. J. Biochem. 5*, 415–421.

44. Lyman, R.L., Sheehan, G., and Tinoco, J. (1971) Diet and $^{14}CH_3$-Methionine Incorporation into Liver Phosphatidylcholine Fractions of Male and Female Rats, *Canad. J. Biochem. 49*, 71–79.

45. Lindblad, L., and Schersten, T. (1976) Incorporation Rate In Vitro of Choline and Methyl-Methionine into Human Hepatic Lecithins, *Scand. J. Gastroent. 11*, 587–591.

46. Drouva, S.V., Rerat, E., Leblanc, P., Laplante, E., and Kordon, C. (1987) Variations of Phospholipid Methyltransferase(s) Activity in the Rat Pituitary: Estrous Cycle and Sex Differences, *Endocrinol. 121*, 569–574.

47. Young, D.L. (1971) Estradiol- and Testosterone-Induced Alterations in Phosphatidylcholine and Triglyceride Synthesis in Hepatic Endoplasmic Reticulum, *J. Lipid Res. 12*, 590–595.

48. Holmes-McNary, M.Q., Cheng, W.L., Mar, M.H., Fussell, S., and Zeisel, S.H. (1996) Choline and Choline Esters in Human and Rat Milk and Infant Formulas, *Am. J. Clin. Nutr. 64*, 572–576.

49. Rohlfs, E.M., Garner, S.C., Mar, M.-H., and Zeisel, S.H. (1993) Glycerophosphocholine and Phosphocholine Are the Major Choline Metabolites in Rat Milk, *J. Nutr. 123*, 1762–1768.

50. Zeisel, S.H., Char, D., and Sheard, N.F. (1986) Choline, Phosphatidylcholine and Sphingomyelin in Human and Bovine Milk and Infant Formulas, *J. Nutr. 116*, 50–58.

51. Kanfer, J.N., and McCartney, D.G. (1988) Developmental and Regional Quantitation of Glycerophosphorylcholine Phosphodiesterase Activities in Rat Brain, *Neurochem. Res. 13*, 803–806.

52. Pomfret, E.A., daCosta, K., Schurman, L.L., and Zeisel, S.H. (1989) Measurement of Choline and Choline Metabolite Concentrations Using High-Pressure Liquid Chromatography and Gas Chromatography–Mass Spectrometry, *Analyt. Biochem. 180*, 85–90.

53. Kennedy, E.P., and Weiss, S.B. (1956) The Function of Cytidine Coenzymes in the Biosynthesis of Phospholipids, *J. Biol. Chem. 222*, 193–214.

54. FASEB Life Sciences Research Office (1981) *Effects of Consumption of Choline and Lecithin on Neurological and Cardiovascular Systems: Report # PB-82-133257*, Bureau of Foods, Food and Drug Administration, Department of Health, Education, and Welfare, Washington, D.C.

55. Zeisel, S.H. (1987) in *Cellular and Molecular Basis of Cholinergic Function*, Dowdall, M.J., and Hawthorne, J.N., eds., Horwood, Chichester, pp. 709–719.

56. Zeisel, S.H., Stanbury, J.B., Wurtman, R.J., Brigida, M., and Fierro, B.R. (1982) Choline Content of Mothers' Milk in Ecuador and Boston, *New Engl. J. Med. 306*, 175–176.

57. Chao, C.K., Pomfret, E.A., and Zeisel, S.H. (1988) Uptake of Choline by Rat Mammary-Gland Epithelial Cells, *Biochem. J. 254*, 33–38.

58. American Academy of Pediatrics Committee on Nutrition (1980) Breastfeeding, *Pediat. 2*, 1176–1178.

59. Dewy, K.G., Heing, M.J., Nommsen, L.A., Peerson, J.M., and Lonnerdal, B. (1992) Growth of Breast-Fed and Formula-Fed Infants from 0–18 Months: The Darling Study, *Pediatrics 89*, 1035–1041.
60. Foman, S.J. (1993) in *Nutrition of Normal Infants,* Foman, S.J., ed., Mosby, St. Louis, pp. 85–90.
61. Cheng, W.-L., Holmes-McNary, M.Q., Mar, M.-H., Lien, E.L., and Zeisel, S.H. (1996) Bioavailability of Choline and Choline Esters from Milk in Rat Pups, *J. Nutr. Biochem. 7*, 457–464.

List of Attendees

Albrecht, Bernd
Arai, Hiroyuki
Attard, George
Bartholmey, Sandra
Bazan, Nicolas
Becker, Claus
Belding, Mary
Berger, Alvin
Blusztajn, J.K.
Bonekamp, Alice
Bornet, Francis
Brommelsiek, Wayne
Burdge, Graham C.
Cain, Frederick
Canty, David
Carneheim, Claes
Chambers-Dorman, Marolyn R.
De Ferra, Lorenzo
De Kock, Jan
Diehl, Bernd W.K.
Dupont, Jacqueline
Farooqi, Aijaz
Fukushima, Minoru
Geeraert, Luc
Gidding, Curtis
Gotz, Volker
Green, M.K.
Greenspan, Philip
Gross, Richard
Gugger, Eric
Gunnarsson, Torsten
Gurkin, Susan U.
Hagerman, Scott
Hakansson, Ulf
Han, Gyeong Ho
Hansen, Harald S.
Hsia, S.L.
Hunt, Alan
Inoue, Keizo
Jackowski, Suzanne
Karlsson, Anders A.
Koch, Helmut

Kohn, Gerhard
Kronke, Martin
Krzych, Valerie
Lange, Reinhard
Liscovitch, Mordechai
Loy, Rebekah
Marriott, Bernadette
McCaskill, Don R.
McCully, Kilmer
Meck, Warren
Merrill, Alfred
Moser, Ann
Moser, Hugo
Nojima, Shoshichi
Nyberg, Lena
Paltauf, Friedrich
Ponroy, Ives
Rogovin, Jarrow L.
Rousse, Bertrand
Schlegel, Robert
Schneider, Michael
Schroder, Patricia S.
Schwarzer, Koen
Shinitzky, Meir
Smith, Wendy
Suchy, Sharon
Szuhaj, Bernard F.
Thies, Frank
Van Nieuwenhuyzen, Willem
Van Veldhoven, Paul
Vance, Dennis
Vance, Jean
Wendel, Armin
Wiegmann, Katja
Williams, Christina
Wilton, David C.
Witter, Brigitte
Worrall, Charles
Yano, Ikuya
Zeisel, Steven
Zigmont, Randall E.

Index

A

Acetylcholine (ACh)
    and choline status, 71–72, 73–74
    and dietary choline, 11
Acetylcholine esterase, Ach turnover
    marker, 69–73
α1-Acid glycoprotein(AGP), regulation
    of, 3–4
Aminophospholipid translocase, regulator
    of transbilayer phospholipids, 59–61
Aminophospholipids
    assymetry in bilayer, 57
    and regulation of transbilayer phos-
        pholipids, 59–61
Antineoplastic phospholipids
    apoptosis induction by, 36
    and CTP: phosphocholine cytidylyl-
        transferase, 32–38
    edelfosine, limofosine, and miltefos-
        ine, 30
Apolipoprotein E, as cholesterol source, 85
Apoptosis
    antineoplastic phospholipid induced, 36
choline deficiency-induced, 14–16
and endonuclease activity, 14
    prevention by LPC, 36–38
    and sphingolipid biosynthesis, 2, 5, 7–8
    sphingosine induced, 13
Axons
    culture systems for studying lipids
        in, 80–81
    lipid synthesis and growth of, 80–89

B

Betaine, and transmethylation of homo-
    cysteine, 121, 131–132
Brain development, prenatal choline
    and biochemistry of, 69–76

C

Calmodulin, and regulation of myocar-
    dial phospholipase A$_2$, 105–106
Carcinogenesis, inhibition by dietary
    sphinglipids, 5–8
Cell death. *See* Apoptosis
Cell signalling, sphingmyelin and, 2
Cell suicide. *See also* Apoptosis
    choline phospholipids and, 11–16
Ceramidase (s), 2
    activity and interleukin-1β, 3–4
Ceramide
    and choline deficiency-induced
        apoptosis, 15
    and neurite growth, 87–89
    and sphingomyelin synthase, 13
    and sphingomyelin turnover, 2
Cholesterol
    exogenous delivery to axons of,
        85–87
    synthesis and axonal growth, 84–85
Choline
    deficiency and folate deficiency,
        131–132
    deficiency and homocysteine metab-
        olism, 120–121
    deficiency-induced apoptosis, 14–16
    depletion in pregnant animals,
        133–135
    functions of, 11
    and lactation, 135
    milk as source of, 135–138
    nutritional importance of, 24,
        131–132
    perinatal dietary requirement for,
        131–138
    prenatal status, 71–76
    synthesis *de novo*, 133–134

Choline phospholipids. See also
Phosphatidylcholine; Plasmalogens;
Lysophosphatdylcholine;
Sphingomyelin
assymetry in bilayer, 57
functions of, 11
and signal transduction, 11–14
Colon carcinogenesis, inhibition by
dietary sphingomyelin, 5–8
CTP:phosphocholine cytidylyltransferase (CT), regulator of phospholipid biosynthesis, 23, 32–34
Cystathione synthase deficiency
and proteoglycan matrix, 122, 124
vascular disease and, 117, 119
Cytidine diphosphate (CDP)-choline pathway, and phosphatidyl choline, 23
Cytokine, activation of sphingomyelinase, 2

D

1,2-*sn*-Diacylglycerol (DAG), role in
hippocampus, 70
Diisopropyl fluorophosphate (DFP),
and inhibition of PAF acetylhydrolase, 110–111

E

Edelfosine, antineoplastic lipid, 30
β-Estradiol, effect on phosphatidylethanolamine *N*-methyl-
transferase, 134–135

F

Folate
deficiency and choline deficiency,
131–132
and hyperhomocysteinemia, 119–120
Fumonisin(s)
effect on neurite growth, 88–89

mechanism of inhibition, 87–88
and sphingolipid biosynthesis, 5

G

Glycolysis, and coupling with calcium-
independent phospholipase A_2,
104–105
Glycophospholipids, effect of inhibitors
on neurite growth, 87–89
Growth factor, and sphingomyelin
turnover, 2
GTP binding protein (G-protein),
activation of, 12

H

High-density lipoprotein-2 (HDL-2),
and axonal growth, 86, 87
High-density lipoprotein-3 (HDL-3),
and axonal growth, 86, 87
Homocysteine
atherogenic effects of, 117–120, 126
dietary factors and, 119–120
genetic factors and, 119
control of metabolism of, 120–121
sulfation and macromolecular
conformation, 122–124
thioretinaco ozonide and cellular
respiration, 124–127
and vascular disease, 117–127
Homocysteine thiolactone
and conformational changes in
proteins, 122–123
free base, 123–124
toxicity of, 126
synthesis, 120
in malignant cells, 120–121,
122–123
vascular disease and parenteral,
117–118
Homocystinuria, description of, 117

3-Hydroxy-3-methylglutaryl-CoA reductase, inhibition by pravastatin, 85
Hyperhomocysteinemia, and arteriosclerosis, 119–120

I

Interleukin-1β (IL-1β), regulation of gene expression by, 3–4

L

Lactation, and choline depletion, 135
Limofosine, antineoplastic phospholipid, 30
Lipids, growth and metabolism of axonal, 80–89
Lipoprotein phosphatidylcholine, and neurite growth, 87
Lipoproteins, classes of serum, 86
LIS-1 protein, and Miller-Dieker syndrome, 111, 112
Low-density lipoprotein (LDL)
    and axonal growth, 86, 87
    and homocysteine, 122, 126
    and homocysteine thiolactone, 124
Lowe syndrome, and phosphatidylinositol metabolism, 92–97
Lysophosphatidylcholine
    and ET-18-OCH$_3$-induced apoptosis prevention, 36–38
    and PtdCho synthesis, 34
    role in signal transduction, 12

M

Membrane trafficking
    role of phosphoinositides and phospholipase D in, 45–52
Methionine, transmethylation of homocysteine, 121, 131–132
Methylcobalamin
    and homocysteine metabolism, 117

and transmethylation of homocysteine, 121
Methylenetetrahydrofolate reductase deficiency and atherogenesis, 117
    risk factor for hyperhomocysteinemia and cardiovascular disease, 119
Milk, as choline source, 135–138
Miller-Dieker syndrome, and PAF metabolism, 112–113
Miltefosine, antineoplastic lipid, 30
Myelin, and recycled cholesterol, 85
Myocardial ischemia, nature of, 100
Myocardial membranes, phospholipid composition of sarcolemmal, 100–101
Myocardial phospholipase A$_2$
    coupling of glycolysis and phospholipolysis mediated by, 104–105
    nature of and mechanism of, 102–104
    regulation by calmodulin, 105–106

O

OCRL1 gene, and Lowe syndrome, 92–96

P

PEMT2
    regulation of hepatocyte cell division, 25–27
    tumor suppressor, 27
Phagocytosis, and phosphatidylserine, 62–65
Phosphatidic acid
    formation of, 45
    and lysophosphatidic acid formation, 47
    role in signal transduction, 12
    as second messenger, 48, 69–70
Phosphatidylalcohols, formation of, 45
Phosphatidylcholine
    axonal growth and synthesis of, 82–84

biosynthesis of, 23–24
and cell division, 24–25
inhibition by antineoplastic phospholipids, 30–39
LPC regulation of synthesis, 34–35
molecular dynamics of vesicles composed of, 101–102
and signal transduction, 11–14
Phosphatidylethanolamine *N*-methyl-
transferase (PEMT)
and choline synthesis, 133–134
effect of sex hormones on, 134–135
and regulation of hepatocyte cell
division, 23–28
Phosphatidylinositol, metabolism and
Lowe syndrome, 92–97
Phosphatidylinositol 4,5-biphosphate
[PtdIns(4,5)P$_2$]
phospholipase D co-factor, 49–50
roles for, 93–97
Phosphatidylinositol 4,5-biphosphate
[PtdIns(4,5)P$_2$] 5-phosphatasc,
deficiency in Lowe patient
fibroblasts, 92–97
Phosphatidylserine
consequences of surface-exposed,
62–65
measurement of surface-exposed,
58–59
receptors, 64
Phosphoadenosine phosphosulfate,
formation of, 122
Phosphocholine, in milk, 135–138
Phosphofructokinase, myocardial,
103–104
Phosphoinositides, putative functions in
membrane traffic, 50–51
Phospholipase(s) A$_2$, myocardial
and coupling of glycolysis and
phospholipolysis, 104–105
nature and mechanism of, 102–104
regulation by calmodulin, 105–106
Phospholipase C, role in signal transduction, 12
Phospholipase D (PLD)
biochemical properties of eukaryotic,
45–47
multiple isozymes, 46–47
phosphatidylinositol-4,5-biphosphate
as co-factor of, 49–50
prenatal choline status and activity,
72–73, 75–76
putative functions in membrane
traffic, 50–51
putative roles in signal transduction,
47–48
Phospholipase D1, identification and
disruption of yeast, 51–52
Phospholipids
antineoplastic, 30, 32–38
axonal synthesis of, 82–83
measuring transbilayer distribution
of, 57–59
protein regulation of transbilayer
distribution of, 59–62
aminophospholipid translocase, 59–60
scramblase, 61–62
and signal transduction, 11–14
Phosphosphingolipids. *See* Ceramide
phosphorylethanolamine;
Sphingomyelin
Plasmalogens
mediation of ion transport kinetics,
102
molecular structure and organizational dynamics of, 101–102
nature of, 100–102
Plasmenylcholine, molecular dynamics
of vesicles, 101
Platelet-activating factor (PAF)
acetylhydrolase
and apoptosis, 15–16

discovery and classification of, 109–110
Miller-Dieker syndrome and metabolism of, 112–113
structure of intracellular isoform 1b, 110–112
inhibition by diisopropyl fluorophosphate (DFP), 110–111
PMPP, effect on neurite growth, 87–89
Pravastatin
and cholesterol biosynthesis, 85
effect on axonal extension, 85,86
Protein kinase C (PKC; serine/threonine kinase)
activators of, 47
and choline deficiency, 16
inhibition by edelfosine, 30–31
inhibition by sphingosine, 13
multiple isoforms of, 12
and signal transduction, 12
Pyridoxine, deficiency and atherogenesis, 119

R

Reactive oxygen species, and choline deficiency-induced apoptosis, 15

S

Scramblase, and regulation of transbilayer phospholipid distribution, 61–62
Signal transduction
phosphatidylinositol 4,5-biphosphate 5-phophatase and, 93
phospholipids and, 11–14
putative roles of phospholipase D, 47–48
Sphingoid bases
and sphingomyelin structure, 1
toxicity of free, 5
Sphingolipids
and cell regulation, 1–9
and disease, 9
inhibition of biosynthesis by fumonisins, 5
in vivo alteration of metabolism of, 5–8
role in signal transduction, 13–14
Sphingomyelin
and cell signaling, 2–5
cycle, 3–4
inhibition of colon carcinogenesis by dietary, 5–8
occurrence and structure of, 1
synthesis in axons, 82–83
Sphingomyelinase(s)
cytokine activation of, 2
effect of corticosteroids on, 13
effect of tumor necrosis factor (TNP)-α on, 13
effect of vitamin D_3 on, 13
Sphingosine kinase, 2
Sphingosine 1-phosphate
formation of, 2
functions of, 13–14
Sphingosylphosphocholine, properties of, 13

T

Thiolation, of LDL, 122
Thioretinaco, chemopreventative and antineoplastic effects of, 124–125
Thioretinaco ozonide, and oxidative phosphorylation, 124–125
Tumor necrosis factor (TNF)-α
properties of, 14
and sphingomylinase activity, 13

V

Vascular disease, homocysteine and, 117, 119–127
Vitamin D_3, and sphingomyelinase activity, 13

9 780935 315868